NIDATION
A SYMPOSIUM HELD IN HONOR OF
PROFESSOR M. C. SHELESNYAK

ANNALS OF THE NEW YORK ACADEMY OF SCIENCES
Volume 476

NIDATION
A SYMPOSIUM HELD IN HONOR OF
PROFESSOR M. C. SHELESNYAK

Edited by Koji Yoshinaga

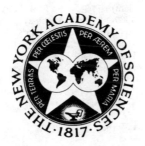

The New York Academy of Sciences
New York, New York
1986

Cover photo: Scanning electron micrograph of the apical surface of epithelial cells on a collagen gel, showing rounded surfaces with numerous short microvilli. In the lower portion of the micrograph the line of attachment of adjacent epithelial cells (arrow) is visible; (×1000). See p. 80.

Library of Congress Cataloging-in-Publication Data

Nidation : a symposium held in honor of Professor
M. C. Shelesnyak.

(Annals of the New York Academy of Sciences, ISSN
0077-8923 ; v. 476)
Result of a conference entitled Symposium on Nidation,
held at McGill University on July 22, 1985, in conjunction
with the annual meeting of the Society for the Study of
Reproduction.
Includes bibliographies and index.
1. Ovum implantation—Congresses. 2. Shelesnyak,
M. C. (Moses Chiam), 1909-   . I. Shelesnyak, M. C.
(Moses Chiam), 1909-   . II. Yoshinaga, Koji,
1932-   . III. Symposium on Nidation (1985 : McGill
University) IV. Society for the Study of Reproduction.
Meeting (18th : 1985 : McGill University) V. Series.
[DNLM: 1. Ovum Implantation—congresses.
W1 AN626YL v. 476 / QS 645 N664 1985]
Q11.N5   vol. 476   500 s   86-23862
[QP275]   [599'.033]
ISBN 0-89766-347-0
ISBN 0-89766-348-9 (pbk.)

PCP
Printed in the United States of America
ISBN 0-89766-347-0 (Cloth)
ISBN 0-89766-348-9 (Paper)
ISSN 0077-8923

ANNALS OF THE NEW YORK ACADEMY OF SCIENCES

Volume 476
November 19, 1986

NIDATION

A SYMPOSIUM HELD IN HONOR OF PROFESSOR M. C. SHELESNYAK[a]

Editor and Conference Chairman
Koji Yoshinaga

Organizing Committee
S. K. Dey, T. G. Kennedy, G. J. Marcus, and A. Psychoyos

CONTENTS

[a]This volume is the result of a conference entitled Symposium on Nidation, held in Montreal, Quebec, Canada on July 22, 1985, in conjunction with the annual meeting of the Society for the Study of Reproduction.

Financial assistance was received from:

- BIOMEDICAL PRODUCTS
- CENTER FOR POPULATION RESEARCH, NICHD, NIH
- DIAGNOSTIC SYSTEMS LABORATORIES, INC
- DUPONT CANADA-NEN RESEARCH PRODUCTS
- FAMILY HEALTH INTERNATIONAL
- HOLTZMAN COMPANY
- MERCK INSTITUTE FOR THERAPEUTIC RESEARCH
- THE ROCKEFELLER FOUNDATION
- SANDOZ, INC
- SANDOZ RESEARCH INSTITUTE
- SERONO LABORATORIES
- SYNTEX CORPORATION
- WYETH LABORATORIES, INC
- WYETH LTD

Preface

KOJI YOSHINAGA

Reproductive Sciences Branch
Center for Population Research
National Institute of Child Health
and Human Development
National Institutes of Health
Bethesda, Maryland 20892

During the Seventh International Congress of Endocrinology held in Quebec City in July 1984, friends and former colleagues of Professor M. C. Shelesnyak gathered to have a small discussion on ovum implantation. A review of the current and past research in this area made it abundantly clear that Professor M. C. Shelesnyak had made many significant contributions to our understanding of such various aspects of nidation as blastocyst-uterine interactions, nidus formation, the endocrine aspect of pseudopregnancy, luteal function in early pregnancy, the mechanism of decidualization, and the preimplantation surge of estrogen. But despite these remarkable achievements we felt that Professor Shelesnyak's contributions had never been formally acknowledged. We—Dr. George Marcus, Dr. Alexandre Psychoyos, Dr. Tom Kennedy, Dr. S. K. Dey and I—decided unanimously to hold a symposium in honor of Professor M. C. Shelesnyak in order to express our appreciation. We formed a committee to organize a one-day symposium to be held in conjunction with the annual meeting of the Society for the Study of Reproduction. Although the one-day limitation restricted the number of speakers, the resulting program was excellent. The symposium was held at McGill University in Montreal, Quebec on July 22, 1985, and its proceedings are presented in this volume. This symposium is an attempt to update our current knowledge of various aspects of nidation. The presentations deal with hormonal requirements for implantation, uterine receptivity for nidation, embryonic signals and uterine response to the embryonic stimulation, a new *in vitro* model for implantation research, application of information available from animals to humans, the role of the epithelium in implantation and uterine receptivity, uterine preparation for decidualization, biochemical aspects of decidual cells, and immunological aspects of implantation and decidualization.

For his contributions to our knowledge on nidation the members of the organizing committee express their deep appreciation to Professor M. C. Shelesnyak. Without his stimulating leadership nidation research would not have reached its current state of development. His assistance in the realization of this symposium is also appreciated. We also thank the participants in this

1

symposium for the contribution of their time and effort to this work. We are also grateful to all of the attendees, who made the symposium successful. The information currently available is far from adequate to be used for improving human fertility or for development of safe and acceptable contraceptive means. It is the mission of those of us engaging in this research to elucidate further the mechanisms involved in nidation because such information is urgently needed by clinicians. Finally, we would like to express our heartfelt gratitude for the generous financial support from the organizations listed on the previous page. Without their support, this symposium would not have been realized.

Introduction

SHELDON J. SEGAL

The Rockefeller Foundation
New York, New York 10036

As we launch this symposium, it is useful to recall the significance of the process of implantation within the broader context of the evolution of the reproductive processes. Restriction of the reproductive rate, along with greater assurance that offspring survive, is a prominent adaptation in the evolution of higher vertebrates. Viviparity, with a sophisticated mechanism for the nidation and nurturing *in utero* of individual offspring, is the ultimate expression of this adaptive process. The physiology, endocrinology, morphology, biochemistry, and immunology of implantation have been studied in great detail, yet key elements of this vital process continue to evade our clear understanding.

From time to time, difficult scientific problems seem to drop from sight, not because the problems have been solved, but simply because they have been moved out of the spotlight of public attention, making room for the more fashionable subjects of the day. Fortunately, there are always the informed and committed who continue to work toward greater elucidation of unresolved questions. Implantation, as a subject of scientific inquiry, has undergone this cycle of events. It is therefore appropriate and timely that we convene this symposium on nidation.

The distinguished organization that Dr. Yoshinaga represents sponsors a workshop on the testis and another series on the ovary each year. Perhaps this symposium will elicit interest in a similar series of workshops on implantation.

It is also appropriate and timely that we pay tribute to one of the field's inspirational figures, M. C. Shelesnyak. Most of us gathered here for this occasion, among Shelesnyak's former associates and colleagues, mark his years at the Weizmann Institute, to which I shall return in a moment. But his contributions to this field predate that epoch by far.

In a letter I received from him recently, Dr. Shelesnyak reminded me that in 1931 he published his first paper on the induction of pseudopregnancy in the rat by electrical stimulation of the cervix. (I was tempted to write back and say I didn't think they had electricity that long ago!) Reflect also that it was Shelesnyak, in 1932 and 1933, who used exogenous estrogens and progesterone to cause decidualization in the immature rat. It was at that early time, over 50 years ago, briefly after the isolation and naming of estrogens and progesterone (in fact, researchers were still debating what to call these hormones), that Shelesnyak first made the observation that the ratio of pro-

3

gesterone to estrogen was more critical than the absolute amounts. Now we can restate this postulate in terms of receptor biology, but the basic principle is vintage Shelesnyak of the Wisconsin era of the 1930s.

Let me quickly move forward in time, some two decades later and a world away, to Israel. In the midst of all her other needs at the time of independence, Israel undertook to establish a premier scientific research institute at Rehovot: the Weizmann Institute. In 1950, Shelesnyak was invited to establish a laboratory there to study problems of reproduction. It was his dream to use this opportunity to create a new integrative discipline that would use the tools of the biomedical, chemical, and physical sciences to study reproduction. And he succeeded eminently.

His laboratory at Rehovot pioneered in the application of interdisciplinary approaches to reproductive problems, a Shelesnyak tradition maintained by his successor, the late Hans Lindner, and by the present leadership of the laboratory. It was a disappointment to Shelesnyak that the name he created for this integrative discipline for the study of reproduction did not endure. What he named the Institute of Biodynamics became the Department of Hormone Research, but the biodynamic concept was built into its very walls, as was the beautiful tile mural created by Roz Shelesnyak in the entrance lobby to depict the reproductive sequence of events.

It was during his Rehovot days that Shelesnyak and his colleagues developed the histamine theory to explain the biochemical basis for trauma-induced decidualization. In a concise, clear, and logical set of experiments, they provided a mechanism for the study of decidualization without the complicating factor of induced physical trauma of the endometrium. With the advent of human *in vitro* fertilization (IVF) and uterine placement of IVF zygotes, uterine sensitization and implantation have begun to move back into the spotlight of public and scientific interest.

With new tools, such as monoclonal antibodies, isolated hormone receptors, and synthetic compounds that are pure progesterone antagonists, we can be optimistic that rapid advances will occur in this field in the years ahead. As we proceed through the papers of this symposium, it will become evident, I believe, that today's progress has been built on yesterday's foundations.

A History of Research on Nidation[a]

M. C. SHELESNYAK[b]

Former head of the Department of Biodynamics
Weizmann Institute of Science
Rehovoth, Israel

It is impossible for me at this time to describe my emotions on hearing of the signal honor you planned to bestow upon me by convening this Symposium on Nidation. It is now almost twenty years since I left the laboratory, the Department of Biodynamics at the Weizmann Institute. As greatly pleased and deeply gratified as I am by this recognition, I am more appreciative of this opportunity to meet again with so many of my friends, students, co-workers, and colleagues, and to meet with younger scientists who find the study of nidation a challenge of exploration and an opportunity for understanding some basic biological phenomena.

At the onset, I want to express my thanks, and pay tribute, to those who had confidence in me and my group, and who made generous, even munificent, contributions for the support of our work and for the facilities in which to do it: early in 1955, Professor E. Rothlin of Sandoz and Professor A. Cerletti, who continued the Sandoz support; later, in 1955, the late Warren O. Nelson of the Population Council, whose work was carried forward by Dr. Sheldon Segal; and, in 1960, Dr. O. Harkavy of the Ford Foundation. The funds made possible not only the research activities of the group, but also the construction of a building to house the Biodynamics Department.[1] I want to thank Sheldon Segal for his continuing support and helpfulness to some of my former students, as well as to other investigators of nidation.

My assigned task is to present a history of research on nidation. The view I shall give will be sharply focused on investigations designed to seek and identify the sequence of events beginning with the arrival of the blastocyst, the fertilized ovum, in the lumen of the uterus and ending with its implantation in the uterine wall, namely of research designed and conducted to arrive at some theory or concept of the mechanism of action. No attempt will be made to describe all of the early research. Frankly, I plan to deal mainly with research carried out by me and my group over a period of about fifteen years, which involved using many avenues of approach in a continuing, concerted, inter- and multidisciplinary effort to understand the blastocyst-uterus inter-relation: a problem of fundamental biological concern.[1]

[a]The author wishes to express his thanks to the generous Grant from Sandoz Inc. to help defray expenses in preparing this paper.

[b]Present Address: 674 Chalk Hill Road, Solvang, California 93463

As I was organizing material for this paper, I became curious about the general development of this field of inquiry. During the golden age of reproductive endocrinology, the mid-1920s to late 1930s, Carl Hartman wrote, "Attention may finally be called to a hiatus in our knowledge of the earliest changes invoked by the impinging egg on the uterine epithelium."[2]

Twenty-three years later, in 1955, at the Fifth International Conference on Planned Parenthood, in his survey of vulnerable points in the reproductive processes, Warren Nelson said of implantation and establishment of the placental attachment, "We know little or nothing of the details of this mechanism".[3] The fact was that very little research on nidation by less than a handful of workers was being done. Then from 1966 to mid-February 1985, there were 594 titles on nidation or implantation in an off-line bibliographic citation list generated by Medlars II, with 152 titles in 1984 alone.[4]

I wrote my fellow participants and asked, "What led you to carry out your research into this subject? Was it a mentor? a colleague? some special research reports of a lecture you heard?" The replies, viewed from the historian's interest, were informative, curious, and even intriguing. I hope they will be told. In turn, some asked about how I became involved; I will try to tell my story briefly.

During my senior year at the University of Wisconsin (class of 1930), I carried out an original research project: postembryonic development of the *Hypophysis cerebri* in *Salmo fario* (Brown trout). This project was under the guidance of Chris Hamre in Professor Hisaw's department (zoology). I still have vivid recollections of miles of paraffin ribbon of serial sections, staining jars, staring fixedly down the tubes of an aged microscope, hundreds of photomicrographs, and reams of literature to read in English, French, and German.

That year, I was in the midst of new discoveries in the endocrinology of reproduction. I am unaware of a good history of that period; some notes on the giants and stars of this drama, however, are available in the second edition of John Fulton's *Selected Readings in the History of Physiology.*[5]

The names Stockard and Papanicolaou, Long and Evans, Philip Smith and Earl Engle, Hisaw, Riddle, George Corner, Allen and Doisy, Courrier, Ascheim and Zondek, and their research stirred overwhelming excitement. Fascinated and enthralled, I spent the summer of 1930 reading and rereading F. H. A. Marshall's *Physiology of Reproduction.* This, the 2nd edition, published in 1922,[6] predated and missed the rapid expansions on the endocrinological side, but it did contain virtually all that was known. The autumn of 1930, as a fresh college graduate, I found myself being interviewed as a possible candidate for the doctoral degree by Professors Philip E. Smith and Earl Theron Engle in the new quarters of the Columbia College of Physicians and Surgeons in New York.

Professor Engle became my mentor, my friend, my colleague, and, at times, my buddy. To him, I owe a great deal. First, he informed me that I had to decide what my research project would be—there were no assigned projects. Second, he gave me some space and cages in the animal room, handed me six female rats and one male, and told me to raise and maintain my own colony. He insisted that every self-respecting reproduction physiologist had to have experience in animal care and breeding. He pointed out the critical need for carefully thought out experimental design to answer the proper question. One should think long and hard before acting. One should always be concerned with the whole animal and its environment, even though studying only a very small part. Lastly, he was adamant about going back to the original sources, the original research reports.

I realize that things are different today. There is an explosive information overload. Editors, confronted with ever rising printing costs, put severe limitations on authors describing the background to research, limiting bibliographic citations to the most current, and suggesting reference to review articles.

The review article can serve a useful purpose as originally conceived, that is, a general survey of the subject with citations of relevant research reports. It is a carefully crafted critical assessment of a group of investigations of the same problem in which the reviewer reveals the consistencies and contradictions, the facts, theories, and speculations. Regrettably, this type of review article is rare today. What appears is a pattern: mainly a telegraphic, telescopic recital, often referring to other reviews (as source material), thus, compounding deficiencies and distortions. It is not that writers of review articles are bad guys, biased, or inept; the system is much at fault.

But I have digressed. My first experiment as a graduate student was to develop an improved method for producing pseudopregnancy in the rat, since it is a useful model. Vasectomized males are efficient, but the method is awkward for use in studies requiring precise timing. The technique described by Long and Evans[7] is only 60% effective. In 1931, I reported 90% success using electrical stimulation of the cervix.[8]

My doctoral research dealt with the infantile female rat.[9-12] The question to be answered was whether precocious maturity, produced by pituitary hormone treatment, developed mature, functional capacity in the uterus. The test model I used was deciduoma formation. This was my real introduction to the wonderful world of deciduomata, first produced in 1907 by the brilliant experimental biologist, Leo Loeb.[13] I found the maturated, infantile uterus capable of forming deciduomata. The research also revealed that the ratio of estrogen:progestogin was critical, not the absolute amounts.[10]

Almost twenty years later, I used the production of artificial deciduomata in the blastocyst-free progravid uterus (pseudopregnant) as a basis for the study of nidation.

The interim of a score of years was an odyssey of research and teaching in biology and physiology, working in a molecular physics lab, trying to study cardiovascular stability and adolescence in boys, working in hospital research units, discovering a naso-genital relationship (and carrying out hundreds of experiments testing reproductive responses to many drugs, all of the data lost when I entered military service), and doing research and training in aviation physiology. I was a member of the Canadian Arctic Expedition (Musk-Ox), a civilian in the Office of Naval Research (USA), and Director of the Washington office of the Arctic Institute of North America.

Late in 1950, I accepted an appointment in the newly organized Department of Experimental Biology at the Weizmann Institute of Science in Israel, and so I finally returned to the laboratory. After organizing the department and starting an animal colony, I turned to the problem: nidation. Several years later, I founded the Institute of Biodynamics, a multidisciplinary group doing interdisciplinary research dedicated to reproduction.[1]

When cogitating ways to study nidation, three general approaches appeared: observational, manipulative, and modeling.[14] Each approach was made from the study of normal, natural gestation; delayed implantation (natural, lactational, experimentally produced); gestation in species with unique nidational characteristics; and ectopic pregnancy.

The observational approach entertains (a) structural states at all levels, from gross to electron microscopic examinations of the uterus as a whole (including its contents), tissue cells, matrix, vascular and nerve networks, and of the fertilized ova; (b) chemical and biochemical profiles of the uterus and blastocyst, including measurement of lipids, glycogen, proteins, polypeptides, enzymes, nucleic acids, electrolytes, and (c) physiological parameters: hormonal status, as well as cardiovascular, vasomotor, and neurophysiological status.[14,15]

Reflecting on manipulative approaches, one could interfere with nidation by altering physiological parameters; by extirpation of various glands, nerves, or ganglia; by administering hormones; by surgical modification of the uterus; by producing special nutritional conditions; by producing generalized stress; and by using various drugs to influence general systemic conditions or targeted genital tract components.

Finally, contemplation of models to disassociate the egg from the uterus suggested (a) a system of free blastocysts *in vitro,* for examination of possible factors influencing the endometrium, and (b) a system using a blastocyst-free uterus to search for factors that induce decidualization and alter the uterine environment from a state of hostility to the fertilized egg to one receptive to it. Decidualization is considered essential to successful implantation. The blastocyst-free progestational uterus was what I chose as a model.

From the time of Loeb's original research, we were aware that production of deciduomas required an endometrium, hormonally conditioned, and stimulated by a nonspecific stimulus. The suggestion of nonspecificity was rejected; we initiated a search for some substance(s) that stimulates decidualization specifically (but, not necessarily uniquely). Because tissue injury is inherent in all methods used to stimulate deciduoma formation, I considered the possibility that some metabolite(s) generated in traumatized tissue would be a likely candidate as a decidua-inducing factor. Histamine was the first metabolite selected for study. Direct intraluminal instillation of histamine, although effective in provoking decidua formation, did not offer useful information, because the act of injection causes some degree of injury as associated histamine release. Therefore, we tested the effect of histamine antagonists on the endometrium of the traumatized uterus. The histamine antagonists were effective in blocking the development of deciduomata.[16–19]

In 1952, I submitted a paper to the American Journal of Physiology entitled "Inhibition of Decidual Cell Formation in the Pseudopregnant Rat by Histamine Antagonists".[15] This was the beginning of a continuing, concerted, multidisciplinary effort to seek the decidual-inducing factor (DIF) and try to understand the process of nidation.

Since antihistamines had various side effects, vasopressor, oxytocic, antispasmodic, parasympatholytic, sympatholytic, and acting as a local anesthetic, these actions, as distinct from histamine inhibition or antagonism, had to be tested. Except for the vasoconstrictor, epinephrine, no locally applied drug prevented deciduoma formation.[20]

Ergotoxine, however, prevented decidualization when administered intraperitoneally. The action differed from histamine blockage; the ergot alkaloid terminated pseudopregnancy and established estrus. The drug also terminated pregnancy. Exploration of the mechanism of action eventually revealed the drug as an effective blocker of prolactin release.[21-42]

It was my good fortune to be invited, a few years later, in 1956, to the Laurentian Hormone Conference to present a report on investigations of ovum implantation. At that time, I made a schema to postulate some pathways of decidual induction, maintenance, and inhibition of deciduomata[14] (FIG. 1). I made some interesting, but unclear observations: (a) There were discrete decidual nuclei (or nodes), in spite of the fact that the entire luminal endometrum was stimulated. These nuclei were spaced about evenly. (b) We observed an asymmetrical response of the bicornuate uterus. One horn was in estrus; the other horn, the contralateral horn, was a massive deciduoma. (c) Atropinization prevented the action of ergotoxine. (d) We observed suggestions (suggestive evidence or nuances), of an immune reaction in the induction of decidualization.

Around 1956, my first graduate student, now Professor Peretz Kraicer, joined me and my loyal, dedicated, and superb assistant and animal caretaker, Shalom Yosef, who had been with me from the first days. Others, students and visiting scientists, followed.[d]

On the assumption that histamine was a decidual-inducing factor, we postulated that exogenous histamine would provoke decidualization. And so we first tested histamine, *per se*, and second, the effectiveness of histamine-releasers (of which BW 48/80, Burroughs Wellcome, was the most active available). Both substances produced deciduomata, but the effective doses were too toxic to allow these substances as useful tools in experimental methods.[43,44]

To pursue this problem, it was essential to find a means of inducing decidualization free of direct uterine contact and probable injury. A Prince of Serendip came to our rescue. While investigating the effect of systemically injected antihistamines, we observed what appeared to be a paradox; namely, one of the antihistamines provoked extensive decidualization. This action led to testing whether the drug, pyrathiazine, was acting initially as a histamine-releaser.[45] This is a reaction known to take place with some antihistamines.

We tested this hypothesis by prolonged treatment of rats with pyrathiazine

[d] See appendix.

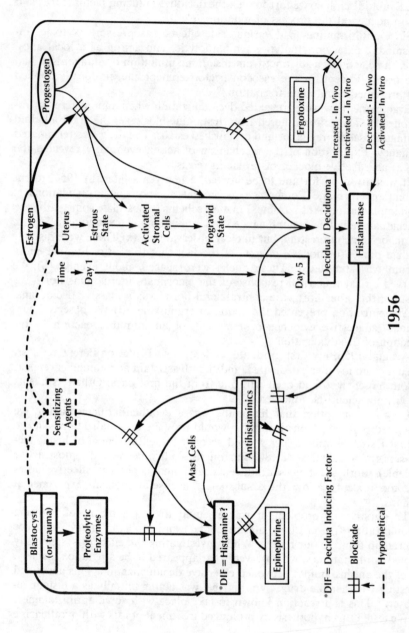

FIGURE 1. Schema of postulated pathways of decidua induction, maintenance, and inhibition.[14]

to see whether the animals would become depleted of their histamine stores. The state of depletion was tested by administering lethal doses of (another) histamine-releaser, BW 48/80. The prolonged pyrathiazine treatment protected the animals from the lethal dose of 48/80, because there was no histamine to release.[46] The pyrathiazine-treated, histamine-depleted rat failed to produce deciduoma, and it also failed to achieve successful nidation and pregnancy.[47]

We now had a fine research tool to use for determining the time of optimal (or maximal) sensitivity to decidualization in the progravid uterus. It was more precise than trauma with its attendant tissue injury.[47] This nontraumatic and noninvasive method also allowed the critical examination of tissue and cellular, as well as biochemical, activity of the uterus from the onset of decidualization to the completed deciduoma.[48-55]

During a sabbatical leave spent in Professor Zuckerman's department in Birmingham, England, I was fortunate that a young Columbia University medical student, Theodore Johnson, was there too and became my co-worker. Thinking about the histamine role in nidation, we considered the various relations between the histamine and endocrine-reproductive system; hypothyroid activity was associated with a decrease in histamine and hyperthyroid with an increase. We considered rapid depletion of histaminase depots following adrenalectomy and hypophysectomy, decidua and histaminase secretion, estrogen and histaminase activation, progresterone and histaminase inactivation, estrogen depletion of mast cells, and the similarity of the initial reactions of the uterus to estrogen with those to histamine, namely water imbibition, increased permeability, and electrolyte shifts. All this information suggested that the initial phase of estrogenic activity paralleled histamine action, and therefore, estrogen action could be considered as histamine-releasing. To test this, we gave a single injection of estrogen (in an amount too small to inhibit progesterone) to a pseudopregnant rat to see whether decidualization would occur. It did. Moreover, antihistamines inhibited the estrogen-induced decidualization.[56] At the time, our attempts to measure histamine content of the uterus gave equivocal results. A few months later, as a guest of Professor Marius Tausk and Dr. G. A. Overbeek, at the Physiological Pharmacological Laboratory of Organon, Oss, Holland, we showed that the uterine content and concentration of histamine was markedly reduced during the 96th to 120th hours after coition.[57] This is the time of ovum implantation.

We also found that natural estrogens reduced histamine content and concentration of the uteri of spayed rats.[58] Comparable findings were reported independently by Spaziani and Szego.[59]

To determine the time of maximum sensitivity to decidual induction in our earlier experiments,[60,61] we found the peak sensitivity on day L_4 of pseudopregnancy, about the same as observed during normal gestation.[62,63] (In our laboratory we designate the day of pseudopregnancy as L_0, L_1, L_2, et cetera, L_0 being the day that pseudopregnancy is provoked. For pregnancy, L_0 is the day of insemination.) This sharply delimited period, coupled with observations of estrogen-histamine interactions suggested to us the existence of an ovarian-estrogen spurt or surge around the time of maximal sensitivity.[64]To test this, we removed the postulated source of estrogen by ovariectomy and, alternatively, used a pharmacological anti-estrogen (MER-25) before day L_3 of pregnancy. Each measure was successful in preventing implantation of the ovum. The same treatments to pseudopregnant rats, which were stimulated to decidualize, prevented decidualization. As counterpart, giving exogenous estrogen of day L_4 to animals treated similarly, allowed successful implantation or decidua formation, respectively.[64–67]

The pyrathiazine induction of decidualization offered a means to study the biochemical, histological, and cytochemical analyses of trauma-free uteri. Findings reinforced our hypothesis of an estrogen surge. Between days L_3 and L_4 of pseudopregnancy, the nondecidualizing uterus showed conditions suggestive of estrogen action: increase vascularity and edema, increased glandular activity and infiltration by eosinophilic granulocyts, and a sudden increase in DNA synthesis.[48] There was also an increase of uterine mass, of proteins, and of nucleic acids.[65]

It appeared that the estrogen surge created conditions that prepared the stimulated uterus to decidualize. After the stimulus was applied, there was an exponential increase in the mass of the uterus, of protein, and of nucleic acids, an accumulation of RNA, glycogen, and lipids in the decidualizing regions.[54,55]

By 1959, we proposed the following: estrogen of the estrogen surge, secreted by the ovary, released histamine that acted on the hormonally prepared progravid endometrium to induce decidualization and decidual tissue into which the blastocyst could embed. Soon, the validity of this proposition was challenged by evidence that there was an estrogen surge in the pseudopregnant rat, not only in the impregnated one.[64,65] Were the hypothesis valid, surge estrogen of pseudopregnancy should release uterine histamine that would, in turn, initiate decidualization and develop deciduoma. In other words, "spontaneous deciduoma" should appear in all pseudopregnant rats, obviating the need for external stimuli. But, spontaneous deciduomata are rare indeed.[69] Measurement of content and concentration of uterine histamine revealed minimal amounts. We concluded that these small quantities were not released, and the pyrathiazine and trauma-induced deciduomas are results of extrauterine histamine, or "induced-histamine".[67]

We investigated the basis for the different amounts of histamine in uteri of pseudopregnant and progravid rats. Our standard method of producing pseudopregnancy was electrical stimulation of the cervix at proestrus. In these experiments, vasectomized males were mated with females to produce pseudopregnancy. We discovered that the uteri of such sterile-mated rats, which had sperm-free ejaculate, also had a higher content of histamine than the uteri of the electrically stimulated rats.[70] Yet, in spite of the elevated histamine level, and the presence of an estrogen surge, there was no "spontaneous" decidual reaction.[69]

We observed that a nonsteriodal, antiestrogen (MER-25) prevented decidua formation, and the associated increased cellular activity. It did not, however, prevent the other actions of surge estrogen related to histamine release in the progravid uterus.[66] We also observed that intraluminal antihistamine administered before the predicted estrogen surge did inhibit decidualization, but not the other manifestations of the estrogen.[47]

These findings forced us to conclude that decidualization requires both estrogen and histamine. Estrogen, however, does not cause histamine release from an intact uterus, nor is estrogen mediated by histamine. They suggest that the blastocyst is somehow involved in histamine release.

Recalling some earlier experiments, we remembered that when antihistamine was inserted into the uterus of a rat in proestrum, and the rat was stimulated to decidualize on day L_4 of pseudopregnancy, the drug effectively blocked decidualization. If, however, it was inserted 24 hours prior to proestrum, the drug was ineffective.[71] We were led to suspect that the estrogen associated with proestrus played a role in the nidatory process. By testing for the uterine retention of inserted histamine, using tritium-labeled antihistamine, we discovered that the occurrence of an intervening estrus abolished the inhibitory action of the drug by either removal or disposal of it.[72] Because susceptibility to antihistaminic blocking of decidualization was coincident with proestrus and its associated estrogen-stimulated uterine growth, we proposed that the estrogen of proestrus had some special action. This action of the estrogen of proestrus we designated as "priming" estrogen; the action stimulated the turnover or formation, or both, of some components of the uterus that bound antihistamine. Thus, the priming action of proestrus estrogen established a potential for decidualization and for its inhibition.[68]

This information permitted speculating on the existence of labile uterine receptors for inducing the decidual reaction. Receptors, which are formed in response to priming estrogen, are stimulated to decidualize by surge estrogen. Studies using ^{14}C-labeled histamine to examine tissue retention gave added evidence, albeit indirect, for the existence of histamine-linked receptors formed by priming estrogen[73] and needed for decidualization.

At this time, a detailed analysis of uterine cellular interactions during progestation and implantation was being conducted. Critical histological and histochemical study of the uterus of the impregnated rat was augmented with autoradiographic techniques to aid in interpreting observations and to trace the origins of various tissue elements.[54] The results of these studies are too extensive for inclusion in this paper, but they warrant being sought in the original. One set of observations, however, merits attention here: the infiltration of the uterus by eosinophilic granulocytes, which is a normal feature of estrus, is dependent upon the priming estrogen, and is greatly augmented by neutrophilic leukocytes following coition.

The analysis of these cellular interactions during progestation and nidation (reported above and see ref. 54) invited attention to similarities between cellular dynamics of early gestation and cutaneous-delayed hypersensitivity,[74] and added to earlier speculations of an immunological component of the processes of decidualization and implantation.[14] In August, 1967, we summarized our concept of

nidation as a sequence of overlapping phases, each characterized by predominating events. The first phase, priming, which includes proestrus and estrus, is characterized by estrogen dominance, which stimulates turnover of uterine components and the formation of new elements, conferring upon the uterus the potential to respond to decidual induction and, as well, vulnerability to inhibition of decidualization. Priming gives way to the second phase, which we prefer to call sensitization. This phase is characterized by coitally augmented infiltration of the uterus by leucocytes and the concomitant accumulation of histamine. The phase is completed by the oestrogen surge which produces the phase of sensitization, and uterine sensitivity is now established. In this stage, the blastocyst enters the uterus, sheds its zona pellucida and induces histamine release, which initiates decidualization. Once decidualization is underway, the blastocyst begins penetration of the uterine epithelium and embeds itself in the nidus. Proliferation of trophoblastic and embryonic tissues has begun with implantation, and nidation is complete.[75] (See FIG. 2.)

It is clear that a great deal of information has been garnered about nidation from using the deciduomata as a model system. Experimentally induced decidualization, as well as decidualization of early gestation, have served to elucidate the mechanism of nidation.

Decidualization has been, and can continue to be, an excellent model system.[76] An excellent analysis of this subject should be called to attention, because it apparently has been almost totally overlooked. *Decidualization: An Experimental Study*[77] was presented in 1960 at the "Colloque Sur Les Fonctions de Nidation Uterine" in Brussels and published in French. In spite of its antiquity, having been written a quarter of a century ago, it merits reading.

Additional research findings led us to elaborate our concept of decidualization:

We believe that, therefore, uterine ability to undergo decidualization is determined by a sequence of events which begins with the action of oestrogen in the cycling rat, causing division of stem cells, the progeny providing precursor cells for decidualization which become competent predecidual cells in synthesizing DNA in response to a phase of oestrogen action during progestation, but without undergoing division. The stimulus for differentiation into the primary decidual cell is mediated by histamine, released by interaction of the blastocyst with uterine elements, or provided by experimental stimulation. The predecidual cell has a temporary potential for transformation and if not stimulated, degenerates within a day or two. The interaction between the blastocyst and the uterus bears features of an immunological reaction of the delayed hypersensitivity type, the sensitization being possibly due to exposure of the uterus to semen.[78]

Final reference in this history brings us to 1970, at the Schering Symposium on Intrinsic and Extrinsic Factors in Early Mamalian Development, where Dr. Marcus and I discussed *Steroidal Conditioning of the Endometrium for Nidation*[79] (FIG. 3). The paper included evidence from cytological studies to support the contention that proestrus estrogen is a determinant of the uterine sensitivity to decidual induction:

Until very recently, our knowledge of hormonal regulation of implantation consisted of essentially only what the hormonal requirements are. The nature

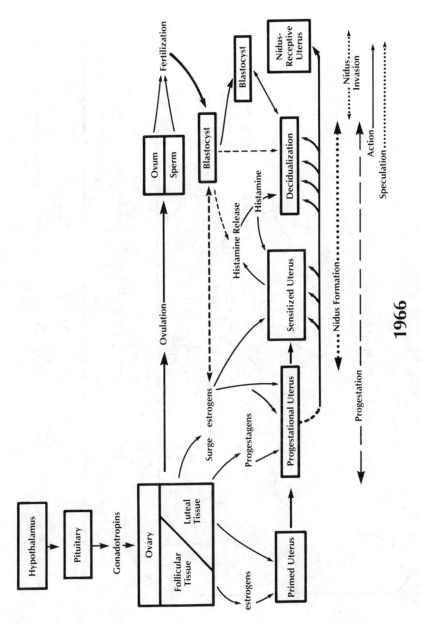

FIGURE 2. Postulated mechanism of nidation.[1]

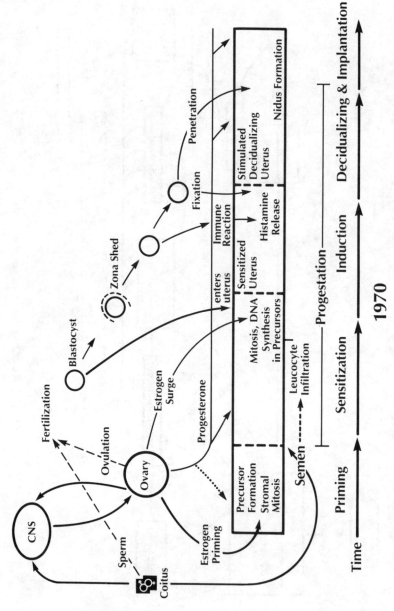

FIGURE 3. Current (1970) concept of the events and interactions in nidation (excluding actions of uterus on ovum).[79]

of the hormonal involvement has been obscure. We are now obtaining the beginnings of some insight into just what is accomplished by the hormones at the cellular level. Conditioning of the uterus for interaction with the blastocyst begins before pregnancy is initiated. The estrogen which is secreted in the preovulatory period stimulates the proliferation of cells of the uterine stroma and also causes renewal of the glandular and luminal epithelia. After a period of exposure to progesterone the responses of these tissues to estrogenic stimulation is altered: the epithelia are induced to secrete materials, which augmented by substances diffusing from the subepithelial capillary bed, may be presumed to stimulate post-blastocystic development; intense proliferation of stromal cells takes place, but in addition, some stromal cells, possibly non-dividing, acquire the capability of transforming into decidual cells upon stimulation—this capability may be associated with non-premitotic DNA synthesis. Both the stromal and epithelial responses are dependent on both estrogen and progesterone. Failure of either response results in the failure of implantation which cannot proceed in the uterus without both adequate secretion and decidual tissue formation.[79]

In opening this historical view of early research in nidation, I stated that my presentation would be largely limited to the research carried out by me and my coworkers. Any misgivings I had at the onset of so parochial a presentation were dissipated while reviewing literature in preparing this talk. In spite of many reviews, proceedings of conferences, workshops, symposia, and numerous research reports since 1960, there has been less than adequate attention paid to the specific, extensive, and detailed research reports originating from the Biodynamics group. It is true we provoked a good deal of controversy and disagreement, which was all to the good, but the neglect (whether benign, deliberate, or careless) does no credit to the investigation of the mechanism of nidation. There is one article that I authored that is the singularly most cited of our work, and I confess that it infuriates me. It is an article invited by the editor of *Endeavour,* an attractive British journal along the lines of *Scientific American.* It has become a source! I hope this presentation of the early history of research in nidation will encourage the reader to go back to the original reports, not only ours,[80–104] so that the concepts and theories developed from the investigations can form a framework for incorporation of the much fine work you, my colleagues, have done and are continuing to do. I look to Dr. Marcus to bring the 1970 proposition up to date when he closes this symposium.

I want to stress, emphatically, that my focused historical picture, with its deliberately delimited view, should in no way be construed as a lack of appreciation of all of the other investigators' research work. Alex Psychoyos has written a fine review of ovum implantation, superior to any other I know.[105]

Finally, I am happy to thank all my former students and coworkers (professional, administrative, technical, and general support staff) for their help. You can recognize many by perusing the authors of our publications. But two special friends, whose names do not appear, deserve my best thanks. Mrs. Rina Yitzchaki was the administrative officer of the Biodynamics Department; her skill and dedication made molehills out of the mountains of researchers' requests and requirements. Very special thanks go to Mr. Shalom Yosef, who was my devoted and talented assistant from the first days. He was the moving spirit in developing and maintaining a superb animal colony; he gave leadership to the support staff and infinite patience and wisdom to my students.

As I dealt with the past, other speakers will deal with the present, and all of us should think of the future.

Permit me to quote the closing sentence of a lecture I gave in 1964 in London at the Second International Congress of Endocrinology: "We cannot move ahead without knowing where we are; we cannot know where we are without knowing where we were." [104]

REFERENCES

1. SHELESNYAK, M. C. 1966. Biodynamics and the population explosion. Ariel **13**: 21-33.
2. HARTMAN, C. G. 1932. Ovulation and the transport and viability of ova and sperm in the female genital tract. *In* Sex and Internal Secretions. E. Allen, Ed.: 647-733 (p. 693). Williams and Wilkins, Baltimore, Md.
3. NELSON, W. O. 1955. Survey of studies relating to vulnerable points in the reproductive processes. *In* Rept. Proc. Fifth International Conference on Planned Parenthood: 157-163 (p. 162). International Planned Parenthood Federation, London, UK.
4. MEDLARS II. National Library of Medicine. National Institute of Health. Bethesda, Md.
5. FULTON, J. F. 1966. Selected Readings in the History of Physiology. 2nd edit. (Completed by L. G. Wilson). C. C. Thomas. Springfield, Ill.
6. MARSHALL, F. H. A. 1922. Physiology of Reproduction. 2nd edit. Longmans. Green, London, UK.
7. LONG, J. A. & H. M. EVANS. 1922. The oestrus cycle in the rat and its associated phenomena. Mem. University California. **6**: 1-148.
8. SHELESNYAK, M. C. 1931. The induction of pseudopregnancy in the rat by means of electrical stimulation. Anat. Rec. **49**: 179-183.
9. SHELESNYAK, M. C. 1931. The production of placentomata in young rats following gonadal stimulation with pituitary implants. Am. J. Physiol. **98**: 387-393.
10. SHELESNYAK, M. C. 1933. The production of deciduomata in spayed immature rats after oestrin and progestin treatment. Anat. Rec. **56**: 211-217.
11. SHELESNYAK, M. C. 1933. The production of deciduomata immature rats by pregnancy urine treatment. A demonstration of the functional capacity of induced corpora lutea in the infantile rat. Am. J. Physiol. **104**: 693-699.
12. SHELESNYAK, M. C. 1933. The production of deciduomata in immature rats by pituitary treatment. Endocrinology **17**: 578-582.
13. LOEB, L. 1907. Ueber die experimentelle Erzeugung von Knoten von Deciduagewebe in dem Uterus des Meerschweinchens nach stattgefundener Copulation. Zbl. Allg. Path. U. Path. Anat. **18**: 563-565.
14. SHELESNYAK, M. C. 1957. Some experimental studies on the mechanism of ova-implantation in the rat. Recent Prog. Horm. Rex. **13**: 269-322.
15. ECKSTEIN, P., M. C. SHELESNYAK & E. C. AMOROSO. 1959. A survey of the physiology of ovum-implantation in mammals. Mem. Soc. Endocrinol. **6**: 3-12.
16. SHELESNYAK, M. C. 1952. The inhibition of decidual cell reaction (deciduomata) in the rat by local action of diphenhydramine (benadryl). Bull. Res. Counc. Isr. **2**: 74.
17. SHELESNYAK, M. C. 1952. Inhibition of the decidual cell reaction in the pseudopregnant rat by histamine antagonists. Am. J. Physiol. **170**: 522-527.
18. SHELESNYAK, M. C. 1952. Inhibition of deciduoma formation by antihistaminic agents. Bull. Res. Counc. Isr. **2**: 202.

19. SHELESNYAK, M. C. 1954. Comparative effectiveness of antihistamines in suppression of the decidual cell reaction in pseudopregnant rat. Endocrinology **54:** 396-401.
20. SHELESNYAK, M. C. 1954. The action of selected drugs on deciduoma formation. Endocrinology **55:** 85-89.
21. SHELESNYAK, M. C. 1954. Reversal of ergotoxine inhibition of deciduoma with minimum progesterone dose in the spayed pseudopregnant rat. Proc. Soc. Exp. Biol. Med. **87:** 377-378.
22. SHELESNYAK, M. C. 1954. Ergotoxine inhibition of deciduoma formation and its reversal by progesterone. Am. J. Physiol. **179:** 301-304.
23. SHELESNYAK, M. C. 1955. The disturbance of hormone balance in the female rat by a single injection of ergotoxine ethanesulphonate. Am. J. Physiol. **180:** 47-49.
24. SHELESNYAK, M. C. 1956. Failure of adrenalectomy to interfere with ergotoxine-induced interruption of early pregnancy in the rat. J. Endocrinol. **14:** 37-40.
25. SHELESNYAK, M. C. 1956. Progesterone reversal of ergotoxine-induced suppression of early pre-implantation pregnancy. Acta Endocrinol. (Copenhagen) **23:** 151-157.
26. SHELESNYAK, M. C. 1957. Failure to detect estrogenic or gonadotrophic activity in ergotoxine. Proc. Soc. Exp. Biol. Med. **94:** 457-458.
27. SHELESNYAK, M. C. 1957. Gonadotrophic content of pituitary of pregnant and pseudopregnant rats following single injection of ergotoxine. Endocrinology **60:** 802-803.
28. SHELESNYAK, M. C. 1958. Maintenance of gestation in ergotoxine-treated pregnant rats by exogenous prolactin. Acta Endocrinol. (Copenhagen) **27:** 99-199.
29. SHELESNYAK, M. C. 1958. Action de différents alcaloides de l'ergot sur la formation du déciduome chez les rats en pseudogestation. C.R. Acad. Sci. (Paris) **247:** 2525-2528.
30. SHELESNYAK, M. C. 1961. Further studies on the mechanism of ergocornine (exotoxine) interference with hormonal requirements for decidualization and nidation. Bull. Soc. Roy. Belge Gynecol. Obstet. **31:** 375-379.
31. SHELESNYAK, M. C. 1961. Fertility control in rats by ergotoxine and by ergocornine treatment during progestation. First International Congress of Endocrinology, Copenhagen. Acta Endocrinol. (Copenhagen) Suppl. **51:** 677.
32. CARLSEN, R. A., G. H. ZEILMAKER & M. C. SHELESNYAK. 1961. Termination of early (pre-nidation) pregnancy in the mouse by single injection of ergocornine methanesulphonate. J. Reprod. Fertil. **2:** 369-373.
33. SHELESNYAK, M. C. & A. BARNEA. 1963. Studies on the mechanism of ergocornine (ergotoxine) interference with decidualization and nidation. II. Failure of topical application of ergocornine to reveal the site of action of the alkaloid. Acta Endocrinol. (Copenhagen) **43:** 469-476.
34. SHELESNYAK, M. C., B. LUNENFELD & B. HONIG. 1963. Studies on the mechanism of ergocornine interference with decidualization and nidation. III. Urinary steroids after administration of ergocornine to women. Life Sci. **1:** 73-79.
35. KRAICER, P. F. & M. C. SHELESNYAK. 1964. Studies on the mechanism of nidation. IX. Analysis of the responses to ergocornine—an inhibitor of nidation. J. Reprod. Fertil. **8:** 225-233.
36. KRAICER, P. F. & M. C. SHELESNYAK. 1965. Studies on the mechanism of nidation. XVI. Induction of oestrus by suppression of progesterone secretion by ergocornine. Acta Endocrinol. (Copenhagen) **49:** 209-304.
37. KRAICER, P. F. & M. C. SHELESNYAK. 1965. Studies on the mechanism of nidation. XIII. The relationship between chemical structure and biodynamic activity of certain ergot alkaloids. J. Reprod. Fertil. **10:** 221-226.
38. KISCH, E. S. & M. C. SHELESNYAK. 1965. Studies on the mechanism of nidation. XVIII. Influence of liver on the action of ergocornine in interrupting nidation and progestation. J. Reprod. Fertil. **11:** 117-126.
39. LOBEL, B. L., M. C. SHELESNYAK & L. TIC. 1966. Studies on the mechanism of nidation. XIX. Histochemical changes in the ovaries of pregnant rats following ergocornine. J. Reprod. Fertil. **11:** 339-348.
40. VARAVUDHI, P., B. L. LOBEL & M. C. SHELESNYAK. 1966. Studies on the mechanism of nidation. XXIII. Effect of ergocornine in pregnant rats during experimentally induced delayed nidation. J. Endocrinol. **34:** 425-430.

41. LINDNER, H. R. & M. C. SHELESNYAK. 1967. Effect of ergocornine on ovarian synthesis of progesterone and 20-hydroxypregn-1-en-one in the pseudopregnant rat. Acta Endocrinol. (Copenhagen) **56:** 27-34.

42. KISCH, E. S. & M. C. SHELESNYAK. 1968. Studies on the mechanism of nidation. XXXI. Failure of ergocornine to interrupt gestation in the rat in the presence of foetal placenta. J. Reprod. Fertil. **15:** 401-407.

43. KRAICER, P. F. & M. C. SHELESNYAK. 1959. Induction of deciduomata in the pseudopregnant rat by systemic administration of histamine and histamine-releasers. J. Endocrinol. **17:** 324-328.

44. SHELESNYAK, M. C. & P. F. KRAICER. 1959. La pyrathiazine est un antihistaminique capable de provoquer le déciduome utérin par libération de'histamine dans l'organisme. C.R. Acad. Sci. (Paris) **248:** 2126.

45. MARCUS, G. J., P. F. KRAICER & M. C. SHELESNYAK. 1963. Studies on the mechanism of decidualization. II. The histamine-releasing action of pyrathiazine. J. Reprod. Fertil. **5:** 409-415.

46. KRAICER, P. F., G. J. MARCUS & M. C. SHELESNYAK. 1963. Studies on the mechanism of decidualization. III. Decidualization in the histamine depleted rat. J. Reprod. Fertil. **5:** 417-421.

47. SHELESNYAK, M. C. & P. F. KRAICER. 1961. A physiological method for inducing experimental decidualization of the rat uterus: standardization and evaluation. J. Reprod. Fertil. **2:** 438-446.

48. LOBEL, B. L., L. TIC & M. C. SHELESNYAK. 1965. Studies on the mechanism of nidation. XVII. Histochemical analysis of decidualization in the rat. Part 1. Framework: Oestrous cycle and pseudopregnancy. Acta Endocrinol. (Copenhagen) **50:** 452-468.

49. LOBEL, B. L., L. TIC & M. C. SHELESNYAK. 1965. Studies on the mechanism of nidation. XVII. Histochemical analysis of decidualization in the rat. Part 2. Induction. Acta Endocrinol. **50:** 469-485.

50. LOBEL, B. L., L. TIC & M. C. SHELESNYAK. 1965. Studies on the mechanism of nidation. XVII. Histochemical analysis of decidualization in the rat. Part 3. Formation of deciduomata. Acta Endocrinol. (Copenhagen) **50:** 517-536.

51. LOBEL, B. L., L. TIC & M. C. SHELESNYAK. 1965. Studies on the mechanism of nidation. XVII. Histochemical analysis of decidualization in the rat. Part 4. Regression of deciduomata. Acta Endocrinol. (Copenhagen) **50:** 537-559.

52. LOBEL, B. L., L. TIC & M. C. SHELESNYAK. 1965. Studies on the mechanism of nidation. Part 5. Uterine manifestations of interference with hormonal requirements of deciduomata. Acta Endocrinol. (Copenhagen) **50:** 560-583.

53. LOBEL, B. L., E. LEVY, E. S. KISCH & M. C. SHELESNYAK. 1967. Studies on the mechanism of nidation. XXVIII. Experimental investigation on the origin of eosinophile granulocytes in the uterus of the rat. Acta Endocrinol. (Copenhagen) **55:** 451-471.

54. LOBEL, B. L., E. LEVY & M. C. SHELESNYAK. 1967. Studies on the mechanism of nidation. XXXIV. Dynamics of cellular interactions during progestation and implantation in the rat. Acta Endocrinol. (Copenhagen) Supplement **123:** 1-109, accompanying Vol. 56.

55. LOBEL, B. L., A. WEISSMAN, E. LEVY & M. C. SHELESNYAK. 1968. Studies on the mechanism of nidation. XXIV. Localization of phosphorylase activity in relation to implantation steroid synthesis and myometrial adaptation during gestation in the rat. Int. J. Fertil. **13:** 33-37.

56. JOHNSON, T. H. & M. C. SHELESNYAK. 1958. Histamine-oestrogen-progesterone complex associated with the decidual cell reaction and with ovum-implantation. J. Endocrinol. **17:** 21-22.

57. SHELESNYAK, M. C. 1959. Fall in uterine histamine associated with early pregnancy in the rat. Proc. Soc. Exp. Biol. Med. **100:** 380-381.

58. SHELESNYAK, M. C. 1959. Histamine-releasing activity of natural estrogens. Proc. Soc. Exp. Biol. Med. **100:** 739-741.

59. SPAZIANI, E. & C. M. SZEGO. 1958. The influence of estradiol and cortisol on uterine histamine in the ovariectomized rat. Endocrinology **63:** 669-678.

60. SHELESNYAK, M. C. & P. F. KRAICER. 1959. Détermination de la période de sensibilité maximale de l'endomètre a la décidualisation au moyen de déciduomes provoqués par un traitement empruntant la voie vasculaire. C.R. Acad. Sci. (Paris) **248:** 3213-3215.

61. SHELESNYAK, M. C. 1962. Time limits of uterine sensitivity to decidualization during progestation. First International Congress of Endocrinology, Copenhagen. Acta Endocrinol. (Copenhagen) Suppl. **51**: 547.

62. CHRISTIE, G. A. 1966. Implantation of the rat embryo-glycogen and alkaline phosphatases. J. Reprod. Fertil. **12**: 279.

63. PSYCHOYOS, A. 1961. Permeabilité capillaire et décidualization utérine. C.R. Acad. Sci. (Paris) **252**: 1517.

64. SHELESNYAK, M. C., P. F. KRAICER & G. H. ZEILMAKER. 1963. Studies on the mechanism of decidualization. I. The oestrogen surge of pseudopregnancy and progravidity and its role in the process of decidualization. Acta Endocrinol. (Copenhagen) **42**: 225-232.

65. SHELESNYAK, M. C. & L. TIC. 1963. Studies on the mechanism of decidualization. IV. Synthetic processes in the decidualizing uterus. Acta Endocrinol. (Copenhagen) **42**: 465-472.

66. SHELESNYAK, M. C. & L. TIC. 1963. Studies on the mechanism of decidualization. V. Suppression of synthetic processes of the uterus (DNA, RNA and protein) following inhibition of decidualization by an anti-oestrogen ethanoxytriphetol (MER-25). Acta Endocrinol. (Copenhagen) **43**: 462-468.

67. MARCUS, G. J., M. C. SHELESNYAK & P. F. KRAICER. 1964. Studies on the mechanism of nidation. X. The oestrogen-surge, histamine-release and decidual induction in the rat. Acta Endocrinol. (Copenhagen) **47**: 225-265.

68. MARCUS, G. J. & M. C. SHELESNYAK. 1967. Studies on the mechanism of nidation. XX. The relation of histamine-release to oestrogen action in the progestational rat. Endocrinology **80**: 1028-1031.

69. SHELESNYAK, M. C. & G. J. MARCUS. 1967. On the incidence of spontaneous decidualization in the rat. J. Reprod. Fertil. **14**: 497-499.

70. MARCUS, G. J. & M. C. SHELESNYAK. 1968. Studies in the mechanism of nidation. XXXIII. Coital elevation of uterine histamine content. Acta Endocrinol. (Copenhagen) **57**: 136-141.

71. SHELESNYAK, M. C. & P. F. KRAICER. 1964. Studies on the mechanism of nidation. XI. Duration of the inhibition of decidual induction by antihistamine. J. Reprod. Fertil. **8**: 287-292.

72. MARCUS, G. J. & M. C. SHELESNYAK. 1967. Studies on the mechanism of nidation. XXVI. Proestrous oestrogen as hormonal parameter of nidation. Endocrinology **80**: 1038-1042.

73. MARCUS, G. J. & M. C. SHELESNYAK. 1967. Studies on the mechanism of nidation. XXV. A receptor theory for induction of decidualization. Endocrinology **80**: 1032-1038.

74. WAKSMAN, B. H. 1960. A comparative histopathological study of delayed hypersensitivity reactions. *In* Cellular Aspects of Immunity, G. E. W. Wolstenholme & M. O'Connor, Eds. Churchill. London, UK.

75. SHELESNYAK, M. C. & MARCUS, G. J. 1969. The study of nidation. *In* Ovum Implantation. M. C. Shelesnyak & G. J. Marcus, Eds.: 3-25. Gordon and Breach. New York.

76. SHELESNYAK, M. C. 1962. Decidualization: the decidua and the deciduoma. Perspect. Biol. Med. **5**: 503-518.

77. SHELESNYAK, M. C. & P. F. KRAICER. 1960. Décidualisation: une étude éxperimentale. *In* Les Fonctions de nidation uterine et leur troubles. Colloque organise en collaboration avec la section Belge de l'International Fertility Association. J. Ferin & M. Gaudefray, Eds: 87-101. Paris. Masson et cie.

78. SHELESNYAK, M. C., G. J. MARCUS & H. R. LINDNER. 1970. Determinants of the decidual reaction. *In* Ovo-implantation Human Gonadotropins Prolactin: 118-129. P. O. Hubinont, F. LeRoy, C. Robyn & P. Leleux, Eds. S. Karger, Basel.

79. SHELESNYAK, M. C. & G. J. MARCUS. 1971. Steroidal conditioning of the endometrium for nidation. *In* Advances in the Biosciences. Vol. 6: 303-316. G. Raspe, Ed. Braunschweig, Pergamon Press. Vieweg.

80. SHELESNYAK, M. C. 1960. Nidation of the fertilized ovum. Endeavour **19**: 81-86.

81. SHELESNYAK, M. C. 1953. Influence of post-stimulation time-interval upon effective inhibition by benadryl of deciduoma formation. Bull. Res. Counc. Isr. **3**: 112-113.

82. SACHS, L. & M. C. SHELESNYAK. 1955. The development and suppression of polyploidy in the developing and suppressed deciduoma in the rat. J. Endocrinol. **12**: 146-151.

83. SHELESNYAK, M. C. & A. M. DAVIES. 1955. Disturbance of pregnancy in mouse and rat by systemic antihistaminic treatment. Proc. Soc. Exp. Biol. Med. **89:** 629-632.
84. JOHNSON, T. H., C. LUTWAK-MANN & M. C. SHELESNYAK. 1959. Carbonic anhydrase in the deciduoma of the rat. Nature (London) **184:** 961-962.
85. GREEN, S. H., T. H. JOHNSON & M. C. SHELESNYAK. 1960. The failure of antihistamines to suppress the polyploidy associated with regenerating mouse liver. J. Pathol. Bacteriol. **80:** 181-185.
86. BARNEA, AYALLA & M. C. SHELESNYAK. 1965. Studies on the mechanism of nidation. XIV. The catecholamines content of the uterus, ovary and hypophysis during early pregnancy. J. Endocrinol. **31:** 271-278.
87. BARNEA, AYALLA & M. C. SHELESNYAK. 1965. Studies on the mechanism of nidation. XV. The effect of cervical ganglionectomy. J. Endocrinol. **32:** 199-204.
88. VARAVUDHI, P., B. L. LOBEL & M. C. SHELESNYAK. 1966. Studies on the mechanism of nidation. XXII. Effect of hypophysectomy on induction of decidualization and its regression. J. Reprod. Fertil. **11:** 349-357.
89. BATTISTO, J. R. & M. C. SHELESNYAK. 1967. Novel alterations in sera from pseudopregnant and deciduoma-bearing rats. Nature (London) **213:** 822-824.
90. TIC, L., G. J. MARCUS & M. C. SHELESNYAK. 1967. Studies on the mechanism of nidation. XXX. Selective antihistamine inhibition of uterine response in relation to suppression of decidualization. Life Sci. **6:** 1179-1184.
91. SHELESNYAK, M. C. 1955. Studies on the mechanism of the implantation of the fertilized ovum; a fertility control target. Report Proc. 5th Intern. Conf. Planned Parenthood: 201-205.
92. SHELESNYAK, M. C. 1956. Studies on the mechanism of the implantation of the fertilized ovum; a fertility control agent. Acta Endocrinol. (Copenhagen) Suppl. **28:** 106-113.
93. SHELESNYAK, M. C. 1957. Experimental studies on the role of histamine in the implantation of the fertilized ovum. Bull. Soc. Roy. Belge Gynecol. Obstet. **27:** 521-536.
94. SHELESNYAK, M. C. 1959. Histamine and the nidation of the ovum. Mem. Soc. Endocrinol. **6:** 84-88.
95. SHELESNYAK, M. C. 1959. Mechanism of implantation and its control. Proc. 6th Intern. Conf. Planned Parenthood, New Delhi: 151-154.
96. SHELESNYAK, M. C. 1963. Physiological bases for the control of ovum implantation. J. Reprod. Fertil. **5:** 295-296.
97. SHELESNYAK, M. C. 1963. Interdisciplinary approaches to the endocrinology of reproduction. *In* Techniques in Endocrine Research: 231-244. P. Eckstein and F. Knowles, Eds. Academic Press. New York.
98. SHELESNYAK, M. C. & P. F. KRAICER. 1963. Role of estrogen in nidation. *In* Delayed Implantation: E. C. Enders, Eds.: 265-280. University of Chicago Press. Chicago, Ill.
99. SHELESNYAK, M. C. 1964. The inhibition of decidualization. *In* Proceedings, Symposium on Agents Affecting Fertility. C. R. Austin & J. S. Perry, Eds.: 275-289. J. and A. Churchill, Ltd., London.
100. SHELESNYAK, M. C., G. J. MARCUS, B. L. LOBEL & P. F. KRAICER. 1966. Experimental study of decidualization. Proceedings Fifth World Conference on Fertility and Sterility, Stockholm. Excerpta Medica. Int. Cong. Ser. No. **109:** 39.
101. SHELESNYAK, M. C., G. J. MARCUS, B. L. LOBEL & P. F. KRAICER. 1967. Experimental study of decidualization. Int. J. Fertil. **12:** 391-397.
102. SHELESNYAK, M. C. & G. J. MARCUS, EDS. 1969. Ovum Implantation: Its Hormonal, Biochemical, Neurophysiological and Immunological Bases. Gordon and Breach. New York.
103. MARCUS, G. J. & M. C. SHELESNYAK. 1970. Steroids in nidation. *In* Advances in Steroid Biochemistry and Pharmacology. Vol. 2: 369-434. M. H. Briggs, Ed. Academic Press. London, UK.
104. SHELESNYAK, M. C. 1965. Exploration of biological bases for fertility control. Proc. 2nd International Congress Endocrinology, London, 1964. Selwyn Taylor, Ed. Excerpt Medica. Int. Cong. Serial No. **83:** 1365-1372.
105. PSYCHOYOS, A. 1973. Endocrine control of Egg Implantation. *In* Handbook of Physiology, Sec. 7 Endocrinology. Vol. II, Female Reprod. System P42: 187-217. R. O. Greep, Ed. American Physiology Society. Washington, D.C.

APPENDIX

This alphabetical listing includes students, staff, visiting students, and senior scientists and associates who engaged in research beginning in 1956 through 1967.

A. Barnea
J. Battisto
A. M. Davies
A. Gershowitz
A. Horan
C. Isersky
M. Joshi
A. Kaye
E. Kisch
P. F. Kraicer
S. Lamprecht
M. Lappe
E. Levy
H. R. Lindner
B. Lobel

B. Lunenfeld
G. J. Marcus
J. Meites
M. Pinto
E. Simon
J. F. Strauss
C. Tachi
S. Tachi
L. Tic
P. Varavudhi
A. Weisman
A. Zahavi
G. Zeilmaker
R. Zmigrod

Bibliographic Addendum: Reviews and Conference Proceedings

Inclusion in this list does not imply recommendation by M. C. Shelesnyak.

COURRIER, R. 1945. Endocrinologie de la Gestation. Masson. Paris.
AMOROSO, E. C. 1952. Placentation. In Marshall's Physiology of Reproduction. A. S. Parkes, Ed. Vol. 2: 127-331. Longmans. New York.
BOYD, J. D. & W. J. HAMILTON. 1952. Cleavage, early development and implantation of the egg. In Marshall's Physiology of Reproduction. A. S. Parkes, Ed. Vol. 2: 1-126. Longmans. New York.
ECKSTEIN, P., Ed. 1959. Implantation of Ova. Proc. Congress CIBA Foundation, London. 1957. Mem. Soc. Endocrinology, Vol. 6. University Press, Cambridge, UK.
FERIN, J. & M. GAUDEFROY, Eds. 1960. Les Fonctions de Nidation et Leur Troubles. Proc. Collôque of Sociète National pour l'étude de la Stérilité et de la Fecondité organized in collaboration with the Belgium section of the International Fertility Society. Brussels.
BLANDAU, R. J. 1961. Biology of Eggs and Implantation. In Sex and Internal Secretions. W. C. Young, Ed. Vol. 2 (14):797-882. Williams and Wilkins. Baltimore, Maryland.
ENDERS, A. C., Ed. 1963. Delayed Implantation Proc. Symposium. Rice University, Houston, 1963. University of Chicago Press. Chicago, Illinois.
WOLSTENHOLME, G. E. W. & M. O'CONNOR, Eds. 1966. Egg Implantation. Proc. CIBA Foundation Study Group No. 23. London, 1966. J&A Churchill. London, UK.
DE FEO, V. J. 1967. Decidualization. In Cellular Biology of the Uterus. R. M. Wynn, Ed.: 192-290. Appleton-Century-Crofts. New York.
ENDERS, A. C. 1967. Uterus in Delayed Implantation. In Cellular Biology of the Uterus. R. M. Wynn, Ed.: 151-190. Appleton-Century-Crofts. New York.
SHELESNYAK, M. C. & G. J. MARCUS, Eds. 1967. Ovum Implantation: Its Hormonal, Biochemical, Neurophysiological and Immunological Bases. Proc. Biodynamics Workshop on Ovum Implantation. Weizmann Inst., Rehovoth, Israel. Gordon & Breach. New York.
RASPÉ, G., Ed. 1969. Advances in Biosciences. Vo. 4. Mechanisms Involved in Conception. Pergamon Press. New York.

HUBINONT, P. O., F. LEROY, C. ROBLYN & P. LELEUX, Eds. 1970. Ovo-implantation, Human Gonadotropins and Prolactine. Proc. 2nd International Seminar on Reproductive Physiology and Sexual Endocrinology, Brussels, 1968. S. Karger. Basel.
RASPÉ, G., Ed. 1970. Advances in Biosciences. Vol. 6 Schering Symposium on Intrinsic and Extrinsic Factors in Early Mammalian Development, Venice, 1970. S. Karger. Basel.
YOSHINAGA, K., R. O. GREEP & R. K. MEYER, Eds. 1976. Implantation of the Ovum. Proc. Workshop on Various Methods for the study of Ovo-Implantation. Washington, D.C., 1972. Harvard University Press. Cambridge, Massachusetts.
GLASSER, S. R. & D. W. BULLOCK, Eds. 1979. Cellular and Molecular Aspects of Implantation. Plenum Press. New York.

Role of the Corpus Luteum in Controlling Implantation in Mustelid Carnivores[a]

RODNEY A. MEAD

Department of Biological Sciences
University of Idaho
Moscow, Idaho 83843

Members of the weasel family, Mustelidae, are unusual in that the duration of pregnancy is constant in some species, such as the domesticated ferret, whereas others, such as the mink and western spotted skunk exhibit variable gestation periods due to the occurrence of an indefinite period of embryonic diapause and delay of implantation.[1] Whereas much is known about implantation in mustelids, the precise hormonal control of this process remains obscure.

ROLE OF THE OVARIES IN INITIATING IMPLANTATION

The ovaries of mustelids must be present to initiate blastocyst implantation. Bilateral ovariectomy during the preimplantation period prevents implantation and eventually results in embryonic death within 14 days in the long-tailed weasel,[2] 16 days in the ferret,[3,11] 13-32 days in the mink,[4,5] 4 weeks in the short-tailed weasel,[6] and 24 to 58 days in the western spotted skunk.[7] Intact blastocysts have been recovered from 4 to 10 weeks after bilateral ovariectomy of the European badger.[8,9] These blastocysts were somewhat larger than those obtained from intact females, a phenomenon that has also been reported in other species.[3,6] Ovariectomy at first resulted in increased cell division within the inner cell mass and trophoblast of blastocysts from short-tailed weasels but was subsequently followed by cell death.[6] Such observations suggest that although blastocysts of some mustelids can persist for several days in the absence of ovarian hormones, the ovaries are required for long-term viability of blastocysts and induction of implantation.

The ovarian role in implantation has been studied extensively in the ferret (*Mustela putorius*). In this species, increased uterine vascular permeability

[a] This work was supported by NIH Grant HD06556.

25

occurs in the immediate vicinity of each blastocyst early on the morning of the 12th day of pregnancy, day 0 being the day sperm are found in the vagina, (Mead, unpublished data), and the trophoblast penetrates the uterine epithelium later on the same day.[10] Buchanan[3] demonstrated that bilateral ovariectomy of ferrets prior to day 10 post coitum (pc) prevented implantation, whereas implantation occurred without hormone replacement therapy if ovariectomy was performed on day 10 pc, but the embryos were subsequently resorbed. Wu and Chang[11,12] and Foresman and Mead[13] demonstrated that there was a critical period of ovarian function that occurred between days 6 and 8 of pregnancy. They demonstrated this by ovariectomizing ferrets on day 8 of pregnancy and administering progesterone or progesterone and estrogen. Either treatment was sufficient to induce implantation on day 12 pc. If they repeated these same procedures on day 6 pc, however, implantation (i.e. trophoblastic attachment to the uterus) failed to occur, thus suggesting that the ovaries were secreting something between days 6 and 8 pc that was essential for implantation.

EVIDENCE FOR OVARIAN INTERSTITIAL TISSUE PARTICIPATION

Although the preceding studies confirm the importance of ovarian secretions in maintaining blastocyst viability and inducing implantation, they do not suggest which hormones are involved or where within the ovary these hormones are produced. The mammalian ovary consists of three functional compartments: the follicles, corpora lutea, and interstitial tissue. In mustelids, the latter compartment is particularly well developed and represents a sizeable proportion of the ovarian tissue. Unfortunately the precise function of ovarian interstitial tissue is poorly understood and cytological changes in this tissue have not been well documented in mustelids. In spite of this, changes in the histology of this tissue are not well correlated with any specific reproductive event in the mink[14] or western spotted skunk.[15] On the other hand, ovaries of the long-tailed weasel,[2] short-tailed weasel,[16,17] wolverine,[18] sea otter,[19] and American badger[20] contain extensive amounts of interstitial tissue during the prolonged preimplantation period that begins to degenerate prior to or shortly after implantation. Consequently none of these studies seems to suggest increased secretory activity of ovarian interstitial tissue during the periimplantation period and thus do not implicate this ovarian compartment in the hormonal control of nidation.

EVIDENCE FOR OVARIAN FOLLICLE PARTICIPATION

Ovarian follicles exhibit waves of development and atresia during the period of delayed implantation in the mink,[21] spotted skunk,[15] and European badger.[22] In the latter two species these cyclical changes in ovarian follicles have been suggested to result in the observed periodic fluctuations in estrogen secretion during the prolonged preimplantation period[23,24] and to induce proliferation and keratinization of the vaginal epithelium in the badger.[22] Such periodic increases in estrogen secretion, however, do not induce implantation. Since no one has demonstrated any consistent change in follicular activity that is temporally associated with implantation in any mustelid yet studied, there is no compelling reason to suspect follicular involvement in initiating implantation in members of the weasel family.

EVIDENCE FOR LUTEAL INVOLVEMENT IN IMPLANTATION

The corpus luteum (CL) is the only ovarian compartment needed to produce hormones required to induce blastocyst implantation in mustelids. This hypothesis is supported by two lines of evidence, the first of which consists of extensive anatomical observations in the short-tailed weasel,[16] long-tailed weasel,[2] mink,[21,25,26] European badger,[27-29] European pine marten,[30] American badger,[20] wolverine,[18] fisher,[31] river otter,[32] and spotted skunk.[33,34] The CL and luteal cells of these species, which exhibit embryonic diapause, are somewhat smaller and appear less active throughout the period of delayed implantation than during the postimplantation period. Corpora lutea of the western spotted skunk contain two distinct size classes of luteal cells during the preimplantation period that represent different stages in the differentiation of the luteal cells. The more numerous small luteal cells (12-20 μm) have relatively smooth plasma membranes, rod-shaped mitochondria with plate-like cristae, and some smooth and rough endoplasmic reticulum. Relatively few large luteal cells (20-45 μm), which contain extensive amounts of smooth endoplasmic reticulum that is often arranged in whorls, round mitochondria with both tubular and lamellar cristae, and highly plicated plasma membranes are also present. Coincident with renewed embryonic development, which precedes implantation, one can detect a shift in the ratio of small to large luteal cells, and a few days after implantation only large fully differentiated luteal cells are present.[34] This increase in luteal cell size also results in an appreciable increase in diameter of the CL. The density of luteal capillaries increases after implantation in the European badger, and the central region of the CL, which is avascular during the prolonged preimplantation period, finally becomes vascularized.[35] These morphological and cytological changes in the CL parallel changes in plasma and/or luteal concentrations of progesterone in the spotted skunk,[33,34,36] mink,[37,38] European badger,[28,39] European pine marten,[30] beech marten,[40,41] and short-tailed weasel.[42] Such observations are entirely consistent with the hypothesis that renewed embryonic development and blastocyst implantation are dependent upon renewed luteal activity. Because plasma progesterone levels increase prior to implantation in the spotted skunk,[33,36] European badger,[39] mink,[37,43] ferret,[13,44,45] short-tailed weasel,[42] and beech marten,[40,41] several investigators have attempted to induce implantation in the mink, European badger, ferret, long and short-tailed weasels, and spotted skunk by injecting or implanting progesterone or synthetic progestins (see references 36 and 46 for review). All such attempts have failed to induce implantation to the point where embryonic trophoblast attaches to the uterine epithelium even though some treatments elevated plasma progesterone levels to precisely those in intact females at the time of implantation for periods in excess of 40 days. Progesterone does, however, appear to be essential for long-term maintenance of blastocyst viability.[4,46] The second line of evidence that supports this hypothesis is derived from a series of experiments involving ovariectomized ferrets[13] and mink[5] that possessed ectopic CL as their only ovarian compartment. Such ectopic CL were capable of supporting blastocyst implantation provided exogenous progesterone was present, whereas implantation consistently failed to occur in ovariectomized females or those that were ovariectomized and treated with progesterone that was released from Silastic capsules at a rate that produced plasma levels comparable to those in intact females. These data, taken collectively, suggest that the corpora lutea are secreting one or more compounds which, in addition to progesterone, are required to induce implantation.

It is now well recognized that estrogen is required for induction of implantation in the rat[47] and mouse.[48] Shelesnyak and Kraicer[49] deduced that there was a surge in ovarian secretion of estrogen on day 4 of pregnancy, which set in motion a series of events that eventually resulted in blastocyst implantation in the rat. This surge in estrogen secretion was subsequently verified by Yoshinaga et al.[50] and Shaikh.[51] A similar increase in estrogen secretion during the periimplantation period has yet to be demonstrated in any carnivore (see ref. 24 for review). There is, however, evidence for decreased estrogen secretion for several days preceding implantation in the European badger[23] and spotted skunk,[24] which may account for the decreased height of the uterine luminal epithelium at this time.[52]

In our search for the missing luteal factor, which acts in conjunction with progesterone to induce implantation, we have investigated the ability of the CL of the ferret and spotted skunk to synthesize estrogens.[53,54] Corpora lutea of both species were found to possess aromatase activity, and CL of the ferret contained at least one endogenous aromatizable substrate, testosterone.[55] Thus, the potential for estrogen biosynthesis by the CL of two species of mustelids exists. In spite of this, the preponderance of existing data suggests that estrogens are not the missing luteal factor required for induction of implantation in mustelids, as daily administration of specific antibodies to estrogen, from days 3-13 of pregnancy, failed to inhibit implantation, but was capable of blocking uterine weight gain in anestrous ferrets treated with pregnant mare serum gonadotropin and preventing implantation in rats.[56] Periodic increases in plasma estrogen levels occur during the prolonged preimplantation period and are believed to be responsible for increased stratification in the vaginal epithelium of the European badger.[23] Such increases in endogenous levels of estrogen, however, do not induce implantation in the European badger or spotted skunk.[23,24] Moreover, administration of estrogen and progesterone to ovariectomized European badgers,[8] mink,[4,57] long and short-tailed weasels,[2,58] and ferrets[11,55] have consistently failed to induce implantation. Consequently the combined results are not consistent with the hypothesis that estrogen is the missing luteal factor, acting in conjunction with progesterone, that induces implantation in mustelids. This tentative conclusion does not, however, rule out a synergistic role for estrogen in the development of a suitable uterine environment for implantation, as estrogen is never totally absent in intact females.

If the CL produce all hormones required to induce implantation, what compounds in addition to progesterone and estrogen can it synthesize? We began to answer this question by studying *in vitro* steroid metabolism by quartered CL collected from pregnant spotted skunks and ferrets during the pre-, peri- and early postimplantation periods. Results of these studies were remarkably similar in that Δ^5 isomerase, 3 β-hydroxysteroid dehydrogenase was the predominate steroidogenic enzyme in CL of both species. The rate-limiting step in steroid metabolism presumably occurs after formation of progesterone as less than 5% of the ^3H accumulated in all other subsequent products.[54,59] Dehydroepiandrosterone (DHEA), however, was also readily converted to androstenedione by Δ^5 isomerase, 3β-hydroxysteroid dehydrogenase, but less than 3% of the ^3H accummulated in testosterone. Corpora lutea of the American badger likewise possess the enzymatic capability to form androstenedione and testosterone.[60] Thus, if DHEA was supplied to the CL by other ovarian compartments, the CL could readily produce significant quantities of one or more androgens that might be capable of inducing implantation. Plasma levels of androgens have only been measured during pregnancy in one species of mustelid, the European badger, in which androstenedione varied from 0.05 − 22 ng/ml and testosterone varied from 30-350 pg/ml. Both androgens were nondetectable after ovariectomy, thus suggesting that they were of ovarian origin. No correlation between androgen and estrogen levels were observed; however, concentrations of both androgens were positively correlated with plasma progesterone levels.[61] Because some androgens are capable of inducing implantation in rats[62] and mice,[63] we tested the hypothesis that androstenedione would induce blastocyst implantation in ovariectomized, progesterone-primed ferrets. Androstenedione was administered in 1, 2, or 4 Silastic capsules containing a 10×1.47 mm column of the crystalline hormone. These were inserted subcutaneously along with 4 Silastic capsules each containing a 33×1.47 mm column of progesterone just prior to ovariectomy on the morning of day 6 of pregnancy (day of mating equals day 0). The controls received either empty Silastic capsules or 4 progesterone-filled capsules. None of the doses of androstenedione tested were capable of inducing implantation by day 13 (TABLE 1). Moreover, the lowest dose of androstenedione tested did not interfer with implantation in sham ovariectomized females (group VI). Consequently, these preliminary trials suggest that this androgen is not the missing factor, but larger sized capsules should be tested and blood levels of this hormone measured in intact females at the time of implantation as well as in ovariectomized androgen-treated females to insure that appropriate amounts of this steroid are being administered.

All of the existing data are beginning to suggest that the missing luteal factor necessary to trigger implantation in mustelids may not be a steroid. Nothing is known regarding the ability of CL of any carnivore to secrete compounds other than steroids. Recent studies have reported, however, that CL of several species can secrete other lipids such as prostaglandins. Proteins and polypeptides are also known to be secreted by CL of some species. Relaxin is the best-known proteinaceous secretory product; however, one would not predict that relaxin would promote implantation as it suppresses uterine motility.[64] Therefore, elevated levels of relaxin at the time of implantation should prevent spacing of the blastocysts within the uterus, a supposition that has recently been confirmed in rats.[65] Moreover, administration of relaxin during the periimplantation period disrupted the normal antimesometrial positioning of blastocysts and caused a marked reduction in the decidual

TABLE 1. Effects of Three Different Sizes of Silastic Capsules Packed with Androstenedione on Induction of Blastocyst Implantation in Ferrets Ovariectomized (OVX) on Day 6 of Pregnancy

	Treatment	N	Number of Females with Implantation Sites on Day 13	Size of Implantation Sites
I.	Sham OVX + 4 empty Silastic capsules	3	3/3	7 × 5 mm
II.	OVX + 4 P_4 Silastic capsules + 1 empty capsule	3	0/3	—
III.	OVX + 4 P_4 Silastic capsules + 1 10 mm androstenedione	5	0/5	—
IV.	OVX + 4 P_4 Silastic capsules + 2 10 mm androstenedione capsules	4	0/4	—
V.	OVX + 4 P_4 Silastic capsules + 4 10 mm androstenedione capsules	4	0/4	—
VI.	Sham OVX + 1 10 mm androstenedione capsule	3	3/3	8 × 5 mm

response in rats.[65] But relaxin may not be the only proteinaceous secretory product of corpora lutea, as CL of some species have been reported to secrete oxytocin[66–68] as well as proteinaceous angiogenic factors.[69,70] If luteal cell secretions can stimulate mitotic activity in endothelial cells, it is conceivable that such secretions might also have the same effect on preimplantation blastocysts. Our preliminary experiments indicate that both skunk and ferret CL are capable of incorporating radiolabeled amino acids into several different proteins, which were recovered from the spent culture medium, with molecular weights ranging from approximately 14,000 to 120,000 (FIGURE 1). We have yet to determine whether these radiolabeled compounds are secretory products or cellular proteins that are merely leaking into the medium from damaged cells. We also have yet to determine whether these proteins play any role in blastocyst implantation.

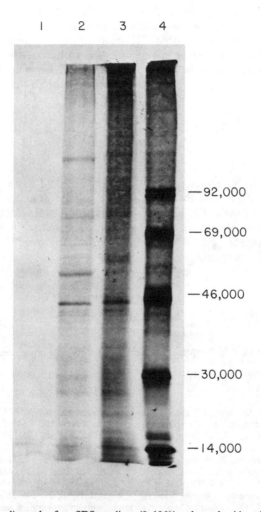

FIGURE 1. Autoradiograph of an SDS gradient (8-18%) polyacrylamide gel showing radiolabeled products obtained from the dialysed spent medium after culturing collagenase dispersed ferret luteal cells in TC-199 with 50 μCi of a ^{3}H-amino acid mixture for 5 hours. Products produced by luteal cells obtained from day 12 pseudopregnant ferrets are shown in lane 1; those produced by luteal cells obtained from day 8 pregnant ferrets are in lane 2; those produced by luteal cells obtained from day 6 pregnant ferrets are in lane 3; and lane 4 contains ^{14}C-labeled known molecular weight standards.

SUMMARY

The studies that have been reviewed in this paper indicate that the ovaries of mustelids play an essential role in induction of blastocyst implantation. Moreover, the data suggest that CL are the primary source of a hormone, which acts in conjunction with progesterone, to initiate the chain of events leading to implantation. The identity of this luteal factor is unknown; however, existing evidence suggests that it may not be a steroid.

ACKNOWLEDGMENTS

I would like to gratefully acknowledge the excellent technical and scientific contributions of Ms. Ann Swannack, Ms. Martha McRae, Ms. Peggy Kintner, and Dr. Kiran Bhatia, Dr. Kerry Foresman, and Dr. R. Ravindra whose fine efforts have contributed so much to our understanding of this topic. I also want to thank Mrs. Pauly Waldron for typing the manuscript and Dr. A. W. Rourke for preparing the electrophoretic gels.

REFERENCES

1. MEAD, R. A. & P. L. WRIGHT. 1983. Reproductive cycles of Mustelidae. Acta. Zool. Fenn. 174: 169-172.
2. WRIGHT, P. L. 1963. Variations in reproductive cycles in North American mustelids. In Delayed Implantation. A. C. Enders, Ed.: 77-97. University of Chicago Press. Chicago, Ill.
3. BUCHANAN, G. D. 1969. Reproduction in the ferret (*Mustela furo*) II. Changes following ovariectomy during early pregnancy. J. Reprod. Fertil. 18: 305-316.
4. MURPHY, B. D., P. W. CONCANNON & H. F. TRAVIS. 1982. The effects of medroxprogesterone acetate (MPA) on gestation in mink. J. Reprod. Fertil. 66: 491-497.
5. MURPHY, B. D., R. A. MEAD & P. E. McKIBBIN. 1983. Luteal contribution to the termination of preimplantation delay in mink. Biol. Reprod. 28: 497-503.
6. SHELDEN, R. M. 1972. The fate of short-tailed weasel, *Mustela erminea*, blastocysts following ovariectomy during diapause. J. Reprod. Fertil. 31: 347-352.
7. MEAD, R. A. 1975. Effects of hypophysectomy on blastocyst survival, progesterone secretion and nidation in the spotted skunk. Biol. Reprod. 12: 526-533.
8. CANIVENC, R. & M. LAFFARGUE. 1958. Action de différents équilibres hormonaux sur la phase de vie libre de l'oeuf fécondé chez le Blaireau européen (*Meles meles* L.). C.R. Seanc. Soc. Biol. 152: 58-61.
9. NEAL, E. G. & R. J. HARRISON. 1958. Reproduction in the European badger (*Meles meles* L.). Trans. Zool. Soc. London 29: 67-131.
10. ENDERS, A. C. & S. SCHLAFKE. 1972. Implantation in the ferret: epithelium penetration. Am. J. Anat. 133: 291-316.
11. WU, J. T. & M. C. CHANG. 1972. Effects of progesterone and estrogen on the fate of blastocysts in ovariectomized pregnant ferrets: a preliminary study. Biol. Reprod. 7: 231-237.

12. WU, J. T. & M. C. CHANG. 1973. Hormonal requirement for implantation and embryonic development in the ferret. Biol. Reprod. **9:** 350-355.
13. FORESMAN, K. R. & R. A. MEAD. 1978. Luteal control of nidation in the ferret (*Mustela putorius*). Biol. Reprod. **18:** 490-496.
14. MØLLER, O. M. 1973. The fine structure of the ovarian interstitial gland cells in the mink, *Mustela vison.* J. Reprod. Fertil. **34:** 171-174.
15. MEAD, R. A. 1968. Reproduction in western forms of the spotted skunk (genus *Spilogale*). J. Mammal. **49:** 373-390.
16. DEANESLY, R. 1935. The reproductive processes of certain mammals. Part IX: Growth and reproduction in the stoat (*Mustela erminea*). Philos. Trans. Roy. Soc. London **225:** 459-492.
17. GULAMHUSEIN, A. P. & A. R. THAWLEY. 1972. Ovarian cycle and plasma progesterone levels in the female stoat, *Mustela erminea.* J. Reprod. Fertil. **31:** 492-493. Abstract.
18. WRIGHT, P. L. & R. RAUSCH. 1955. Reproduction in the wolverine, *Gulo gulo.* J. Mammal. **36:** 346-355.
19. SINHA, A. A., C. H. CONAWAY & K. W. KENYON. 1966. Reproduction in the female sea otter. J. Wildl. Manage. **30:** 121-130.
20. WRIGHT, P. L. 1966. Observations on the reproductive cycle of the American badger (*Taxidea taxus*). *In* Comparative Biology of Reproduction in Mammals. I. W. Rowlands, Ed.: 27-45. Academic Press. New York.
21. ENDERS, R. K. & A. C. ENDERS. 1963. Morphology of the female reproductive tract during delayed implantation in the mink. *In* Delayed Implantation. A. C. Enders, Ed.: 129-139. University of Chicago Press. Chicago, Ill.
22. BONNIN, M. 1964. Contribution à l'étude de l'histophysiologie de l'appariel génital femelle du Blaireau européen, *Meles meles* L. Th. D., Bordeaux.
23. MONDAIN-MONVAL, M., M. BONNIN, R. CANIVENC & R. SCHOLLER. 1980. Plasma estrogen levels during delayed implantation in the European badger (*Meles meles* L.). Gen. Comp. Endocrinol. **41:** 143-149.
24. RAVINDRA, R. & R. A. MEAD. 1984. Plasma estrogen levels during pregnancy in the western spotted skunk. Biol. Reprod. **30:** 1153-1159.
25. ENDERS, A. C. 1962. Observations on the fine structure of lutein cells. J. Cell Biol. **12:** 101-113.
26. MØLLER, O. M. 1973. The fine structure of the lutein cells in the mink (*Mustela vison*) with special reference to the secretory activity during pregnancy. Z. Zellforsch. Mikrosk. Anat. **138:** 523-544.
27. CANIVENC, R. & M. BONNIN-LAFFARGUE. 1963. Inventory of problems raised by the delayed ova implantation in the European badger (*Meles meles* L.) *In* Delayed Implantation. A. C. Enders, Ed.: 115-128. University of Chicago Press. Chicago, Ill.
28. CANIVENC, R., R. V. SHORT & M. BONNIN-LAFFARGUE. 1966. Étude histologique et biochemique du corps jaune du Blaireau européen (*Meles meles* L.). Ann. Endocrinol. (Paris) **27:** 401-413.
29. CANIVENC, R., G. COHERE & C. BRECHENMACHER. 1967. Quelques aspects ultrastructuraux de la cellule lutéale chez le Blaireau (*Meles meles* L.). C. R. Acad. Sci. (Paris) **264:** 1187-1189.
30. CANIVENC, R. 1970. Contrôle de la biologie lutéale chez les espèces a ovo-implantation différée. Colloq. Nat. CNRS. Neuroendocrinologie **927:** 223-233.
31. WRIGHT, P. L. & M. W. COULTER. 1967. Reproduction and growth in Maine fishers. J. Wildl. Manage. **31:** 70-87.
32. HAMILTON, JR., W. J. & W. R. EADIE. 1964. Reproduction in the otter, *Lutra canadensis.* J. Mammal. **45:** 242-252.
33. MEAD, R. A. & K. B. EIK-NES. 1969. Seasonal variation in plasma levels of progesterone in western forms of the spotted skunk. J. Reprod. Fertil. Suppl. **6:** 397-403.
34. SINHA, A. A. & R. A. MEAD. 1975. Ultrastructural changes in granulosa lutein cells and progesterone levels during preimplantation, implantation and early placentation in the western spotted skunk. Cell Tissue Res. **164:** 179-192.
35. SARKER, N. J. & R. CANIVENC. 1982. Luteal vascularization in the European badger (*Meles meles* L.). Biol. Reprod. **26:** 903-908.

36. MEAD, R. A. 1981. Delayed implantation in mustelids, with special emphasis on the spotted skunk. J. Reprod. Fertil. Suppl. **29:** 11-24.
37. MØLLER, O. M. 1973. The progesterone concentrations in the peripheral plasma on the mink (*Mustela vison*) during pregnancy. J. Endocrinol. **56:** 121-132.
38. MØLLER, O. M. 1974. Plasma progesterone before and after ovariectomy in unmated and pregnant mink, *Mustela vison.* J. Reprod. Fertil. **37:** 367-372.
39. BONNIN, M., R. CANIVENC & CL. RIBES. 1978. Plasma progesterone levels during delayed implantation in the European badger (*Meles meles*). J. Reprod. Fertil. **52:** 55-58.
40. BONNIN, M., R. CANIVENC & J. AITKEN. 1977. Variations saisonnières du taux de la progestérone plasmatique chez la Fouine, *Martes foina,* espèce à ovo-implantation différée. C. R. Acad. Sci. (Paris) **285:** 1479-1481.
41. CANIVENC, R., C. MAUGET, M. BONNIN & J. AITKEN. 1981. Delayed implantation in the beech marten (*Martes foina*). J. Zool. **193:** 325-338.
42. GULAMHUSEIN, A. P. & A. R. THAWLEY. 1974. Plasma progesterone levels in the stoat. J. Reprod. Fertil. **36:** 405-408.
43. MURPHY, B. D. & W. H. MOGER. 1977. Progestins of mink gestation: the effects of hypophysectomy. Endocr. Res. Comm. **4:** 45-60.
44. HEAP, R. B. & J. HAMMOND JR. 1974. Plasma progesterone levels in pregnant and pseudopregnant ferrets. J. Reprod. Fertil. **39:** 149-152.
45. DANIEL, J. C., JR. 1976. Plasma progesterone levels before and at the time of implantation in the ferret. J. Reprod. Fertil. **48:** 437-438.
46. MEAD, R. A., P. W. CONCANNON & M. McRAE. 1981. Effect of progestins on implantation in the western spotted skunk. Biol. Reprod. **25:** 128-133.
47. COCHRANE, R. L. & R. K. MEYER. 1957. Delayed nidation in the rat induced by progesterone. Proc. Soc. Exp. Biol. Med. **96:** 155-159.
48. SMITHBERG, M. & M. N. RUNNER. 1960. Retention of blastocysts in nonprogestational uteri of mice. J. Exp. Zool. **143:** 21-31.
49. SHELESNYAK, M. C. & P. F. KRAICER. 1963. The role of estrogen in nidation. *In* Delayed Implantation. A. C. Enders, Ed.: 265-279. Univ. Chicago Press. Chicago, Ill.
50. YOSHINAGA, K., R. A. HAWKINS & J. F. STOCKER. 1969. Estrogen secretion by the rat ovary *in vivo* during the estrous cycle and pregnancy. Endocrinology **85:** 103-112.
51. SHAIKH, A. A. 1971. Estrone and estradiol levels in the ovarian venous blood from rats during the estrous cycle and pregnancy. Biol. Reprod. **5:** 297-307.
52. SINHA, A. & R. A. MEAD. 1976. Morphological changes in the trophoblast, uterus and corpus luteum during delayed implantation and implantation in the western spotted skunk. Am. J. Anat. **145:** 331-356.
53. MEAD, R. A. & A. SWANNACK. 1980. Aromatase activity in corpora lutea of the ferret. Biol. Reprod. **22:** 560-565.
54. RAVINDRA, R., K. BHATIA & R. A. MEAD. 1984. Steroid metabolism in corpora lutea of the western spotted skunk (*Spilogale putorius latifrons*). J. Reprod. Fertil. **72:** 495-502.
55. MEAD, R. A. & M. McRAE. 1982. Is estrogen required for implantation in the ferret? Biol. Reprod. **27:** 540-547.
56. MURPHY, B. D. & R. A. MEAD. 1976. Effects of antibodies to oestrogens on implantation in ferrets. J. Reprod. Fertil. **46:** 261-263.
57. COCHRANE, R. L. & R. M. SHACKELFORD. 1962. Effects of exogenous oestrogen alone and in combination with progesterone on pregnancy in the intact mink. J. Endocrinol. **25:** 101-106.
58. SHELDEN, R. M. 1973. Failure of ovarian steroids to influence blastocysts of weasels (*Mustela erminea*) ovariectomized during delayed implantation. Endocrinology **92:** 638-641.
59. KINTNER, P. J. & R. A. MEAD. 1983. Steroid metabolism in the corpus luteum of the ferret. Biol. Reprod. **29:** 1121-1127.
60. FEVOLD, H. R. & P. L. WRIGHT. 1969. Steroid metabolism by badger (*Taxidea taxus*) ovarian tissue homogenates. Gen. Comp. Endocrinol. **13:** 60-67.
61. MONDAIN-MONVAL, M., M. BONNIN, R. SCHOLLER & R. CANIVENC. 1983. Plasma androgen patterns during delayed implantation in the European badger (*Meles meles* L.). Gen. Comp. Endocrinol. **50:** 67-74.

62. VARAVUDHI, P. 1969. Stimulation of blastocyst implantation in long term hypophysectomized and ovariectomized pregnant rats by means of androgens. Biol. Reprod. 1: 247-252.
63. ROY, S. K., J. SENGUPTA & S. K. MANCHANDA. 1980. Induction of implantation by androgens in mice with delayed implantation. J. Reprod. Fertil. 58: 339-343.
64. DOWNING, S. J. & O. D. SHERWOOD. 1985. The physiological role of relaxin in the pregnant rat. II. The influence of relaxin on uterine contractile activity. Endocrinology 116: 1206-1214.
65. ROGERS, P. A. W., C. R. MURPHY, K. R. SQUIRES & A. H. MACLENNAN. 1983. Effects of relaxin on the intrauterine distribution and antimesometrial positioning and orientation of rat blastocysts before implantation. J. Reprod. Fertil. 68: 431-435.
66. WATHES, D. C. & R. W. SWANN. 1982. Is oxytocin an ovarian hormone? Nature (London) 297: 225-227.
67. FLINT, A. P. F. & E. L. SHELDRICK. 1982. Ovarian secretion of oxytocin stimulated by prostaglandin. Nature (London) 297: 587-588.
68. FIELDS, P. A., R. K. ELDRIDGE, A. R. FUCHS, R. F. ROBERTS & M. J. FIELDS. 1983. Human placental and bovine corpora luteal oxytocin. Endocrinology 112: 1544-1546.
69. GOSPODAROWICZ, D., I. VLODAVSKY, H. BIALECKI & K. BROWN. 1977. The control of proliferation of ovarian cells by the epidermal and fibroblast growth factors. In Novel Aspects of Reproductive Physiology. C. H. Spilman & J. H. Wilks, Eds.: 107-178. S. P. Medical & Scientific Books. New York.
70. HALLE, W., B. SAVIKY, G. HEDER, W. E. SIEMS & TH. ROSNER. 1982. Zur Wirkung von Corpus-luteum-Präparationen auf die Proliferations Kinetik von Endothelzellen aus Kälberaorten in der Zellkultur. Acta Biol. Med. Ger. 41: 1045-1059.

Uterine Receptivity for Nidation[a]

ALEXANDRE PSYCHOYOS

Laboratoire de Physiologie de la Reproduction
Centre National de la Recherche Scientifique E.R.203
Hôpital Bicêtre, Bâtiment INSERM
94270 Bicêtre, France

WHAT IS RECEPTIVITY?

Receptivity is a notion that arose during the last two decades mainly from studies using the technique of egg transfer. It is by definition the unique and exclusive situation in which the uterus allows nidation to occur. In fact, since the initial observation of M. C. Chang[1] in the rabbit, the importance for implantation of a chronological relationship between the age of the embryo and the developmental stage of the endometrium has been shown in all species studied, although the time limits for a successful transfer appear to be extended to several days in some species. In more precise terms, a cooperation between the embryo and the uterus is necessary for egg implantation to occur. This can be achieved only if both partners have reached a certain degree of maturity. The embryo must have reached the blastocyst stage, thus being ready to participate in the nidation process. It also has to be present in the uterus at the proper time, that is, when the endometrium is undergoing the specific changes that are referred to as "phase of receptivity."[2]

In several species the blastocyst can, under certain conditions, wait for receptivity to occur. Thus, in species such as the rat[3] and the mouse,[4] the transfer of an egg to a developmentally younger uterus can even be more successful than when realized under a strict chronological synchronization. On the contrary, developmentally younger eggs when placed in advanced uteri can be forced to accelerate their development in order to be ready at the proper time, as in the case of sheep.[5] However, it can be considered a general rule that beyond the time at which nidation is normally expected to occur, that is, beyond the phase of receptivity, the intrauterine survival of transferred embryos of any stage becomes impossible. The uterus has entered into refractoriness, the state of nonreceptivity.[2,6]

A constant feature of the receptive endometrium is its high vascular reactivity towards the blastocyst stimulus or artificial stimuli.[6,7] This reactivity,

[a]This work was supported by Grants from the Institut National de la Recherche Médicale (INSERM, n° 834014), from the Rockefeller Foundation, and the Fondation pour la Recherche Médicale Française.

expressed essentially by a local increase in capillary permeability, appears to be, in all species studied, the forerunner signal of the nidation process. In fact, increased capillary permeability and decidual differentiation appear to be two phenomena linked to each other. They appear to result from a cascade-like effect involving vasoactive substances such as histamine,[8] and prostaglandins.[7]

Stromal mitosis appearing just before the expected time of implantation in the human[9] and in rodents,[10,11] can be considered also as a correlate of uterine receptivity, together with some other morphological changes such as the basal position of epithelial nuclei, a stromal edema.[2,6] In the rat, an ultrastructural correlate of the receptive endometrium is the presence, on the apical surface of the luminal epithelial cells, of sponge-like structures that can be observed under scanning electron microscopy.[2,12,13] They appear to be pinopodes involved in the pinocytosis and endocytosis phenomena.[13,14] The presence of similar structures is also observed during the luteal phase in the human endometrium at the perinidatory period.[15] A significant thinning of the epithelial glycocalyx[16,17] must also be considered as characteristic of uterine receptivity as well as a reduction in negativity of the epithelial surface,[18] facilitating blastocyst adhesion.

The demonstration of a specific activation or inhibition of a uterine enzymatic activity, which would indicate the receptive period, is missing as yet. Changes in certain endometrial enzymes, however, can indirectly inform us upon the occurrence of the receptive phase. For example, the sudden increase of two progesterone-dependant activities such as the monoamine oxidase (MAO) and catechol O-methyl transferase (COMT) precedes and announces receptivity, whereas estradiol dehydrogenase (DH) activity follows it. In the rat, the endometrial MAO and COMT activities increase sharply on day 3 of pseudopregnancy,[19] whereas estradiol DH increases 16-fold on day 6.[20]

WHEN AND HOW DOES RECEPTIVITY APPEAR?

Until the early 1960s, researchers considered nidation, in an animal such as the rat, beginning when morphological criteria indicated the invasion of the endometrium by the trophoblast or the uterine response to this invasion. This becomes apparent on day 6 of pregnancy, day 1 being determined by the presence of spermatozoa in the vaginal smear. Since then, however, the introduction of the technique of intravenous injection of blue dye has made it possible to reveal a local change in vascular permeability induced by the blastocyst as early as the early afternoon of day 5.[21]

Kraicer and Shelesnyak,[22] using a systemic inducer of decidualization, pyrathiazine, had found in pseudopregnant rats a 4-hr period on day 5 during which this compound was most effective. They suggested that this period could correspond to the one during which the blastocyst triggers its own decidual stimulus. De Feo,[23] exploring further the temporal aspects of uterine sensitivity in this species by using intraluminal inducers, specified that such a period of optimal endometrial responsiveness appears around noon of day 5.

An observation reported by Dickmann and Noyes[24] at this early time in the study of nidation indicated clearly the occurrence of a sudden change by the end of day 5. They showed that 4-day rat ova, transferred to a 5-day uterus and recovered 9 hrs later, were found to be severely damaged. By the end of this day, the uterine milieu appeared to become unfavorable for egg survival. The same conclusion was drawn from experiments in which 5-day blastocysts implanted normally after transfer to 4- or 5-day uteri,[3] whereas if the transfer of 5-day blastocysts was delayed beyond the fifth day of pregnancy or pseudopregnancy, the result was always the same: no blastocyst ever implanted.[25]

The hormonal conditioning responsible for these changes is now well defined.[2,25,26] Briefly, both the receptive phase and the nonreceptive state follow a precise time course after the administration of a minute amount of estrogen. Such an estrogen effect, however, requires a priming of the endometrium by progesterone for about 48 hours. This priming, therefore, first establishes a prereceptive neutral state. During this state, the uterus shows a suboptimal sensitivity for the decidual reaction as well as conditions allowing the blastocyst to survive, but in dormancy. Estrogen, when acting on this neutral state, induces, by 36 hrs, a state of refractoriness. During the latter state, the endometrium is no longer capable of decidual response, and the uterine environment becomes hostile to unimplanted ova. The short phase of receptivity appears as a transient event, however, midway between the neutral and the refractory states. In the pregnant or pseudopregnant rat, the 48-hr priming of the endometrium by progesterone seems to start by the evening of day 2 and is completed by the evening of day 4. If estrogen is also available at the latter time, the receptive phase appears around noon of day 5, followed by the nonreceptive state on day 6.

Progesterone priming for a minimum of about 48 hrs was found in ovariectomized rats to increase the estradiol receptor concentration in the stromal component of the endometrium.[27] In the rat, a similar increase in the stroma cells (and decrease in the epithelium) of the estradiol receptor has also been observed during the first days of pseudopregnancy.[28] Progesterone priming by increasing the amount of estradiol binding sites of the stroma cells enhances their responsiveness to estrogen and redirects the effects of this hormone from the epithelium to the stroma. This change in estrogen action is well shown in the rat and the mouse by the different hormonal regulation of mitosis in the two endometrial tissues.[10,11]

The specific factors, permissive or inhibitory, which are involved in the manifestation of uterine receptivity remain almost unknown. Glasser and McCormack[29] investigated, at the molecular level, the availability of RNA initiation sites in uterine chromatin prepared from hormonally treated ovariectomized rats. They found that progesterone priming for 3 days increased by 500% the number of RNA polymerase binding sites available for the initiation of RNA synthesis, whereas a single dose of estradiol given after the progesterone priming resulted in a rapid decrease in the number of RNA initiation sites within 4 hours. Estrogen that induces receptivity appears, therefore, to restrict gene expression and to alter, at least quantitatively, progesterone-induced transcription. Which proteins are synthesized or repressed by these events remains an exciting task for further studies.

Maintenance of the uterus in the neutral or the refractory nonreceptive states requires a continuity of progesterone administration. Progesterone arrest for a period of 48 hrs returns the uterus to a condition permitting the renewal of its progestational potential.[2,26,30] Why and how are questions that also remain unanswered for the present.

CAN THE RECEPTIVE PHASE BE ENLARGED OR DISPLACED?

A shift of the receptive phase occurs naturally during lactation or experimentally in species such as the rat, where an occasional delay in nidation occurs. In most cases a temporal absence of estrogen is responsible for this phenomenon, whereas the progesterone priming is already assured. The possibility may exist, however, where a shift in progesterone priming may also displace the phase of receptivity, whereas the estrogen presence is assured.

In a series of experiments, the results of which will be reported in detail elsewhere, we used the compound RU 486 to induce such a shift of progesterone priming. This compound 17β-hydroxy-11β-(4-dimethylaminophenyl)-17α-(1-propynyl) estra-4,9-dien-3-one is a potential synthetic antiprogestin, devoid of estrogenic activity, showing a great affinity for glucocorticoid and progestin receptors.[31]

Different doses of RU 486 were, therefore, injected subcutaneously to rats on day 1 or 2 of pregnancy. On day 2 one of the oviducts was removed in order to obtain a "sterile" horn and 100 μl of sesame oil injected into this horn on day 6 or 7 postcoitum. The animals thus treated were sacrificed on day 10 or 11.

Treatment by RU 286 on day 1 of pregnancy was found to increase 5-6-fold the percentage of animals showing decidualization and from 190-655 mg the mean weight of the decidualized horns after the intraluminal oil injection on day 7. Obviously, under the above conditions, the antiprogestin appears to postpone the sensitive period and to allow decidualization to be induced at a moment when the uterus, under normal conditions, should be in refractoriness. Furthermore, preliminary results have shown us that under such a treatment by RU 486, the uterus permits also the survival and implantation of blastocysts transferred into a "sterile" horn on days 6 or 7 of pregnancy.

Increasing doses of RU 486 administered on day 2, however, show a strong antifertility effect, reducing the nidation rate to zero (TABLE 1). Our current studies show us that this latter effect results from a deleterious effect of RU 486 on egg survival, similar to the effect of antiprogesterone monoclonal antibodies observed in mice.[32]

TABLE 1. Effect of the Antiprogestin RU 486 on Nidation and Decidualization

| Treatment | | Number of animals | Nidation Rate | | Decidualization[a] | |
Dose mg/kg subcutaneously	Day		Percentage of animals with nidations	Ratio nidations/ corpus lutea	Percentage of animals with decidualization	Coefficient of decidualization
2.5	1	7	71	0.85	100	0.57
5	1	8	58	0.33	87	0.67
10	1	11	27	0.5	73	0.68
10	2	6	16	0.28	33	0.37
10	1 + 2	8	0	0	0	0
Control	—	18	100	0.98	14	0.25

[a]Induced by intraluminal oil on day 7 (see text).

CONCLUSIONS

Some morphological and biochemical uterine changes may serve as markers for uterine receptivity, for example, the presence of pinopodes on the apical surface of the luminal epithelium or the increased COMT activity in the endometrium. The antiprogesterone RU 486 given on day 1 of pregnancy extends the receptive phase beyond its normal timing and postpones the establishment of the uterine refractoriness. This same treatment shows a strong antifertility effect by affecting egg survival.

ACKNOWLEDGMENTS

We thank Dr. D. Philibert and Dr. R. Deraedt of the Centre de Recherche Roussel UCLAF for providing the RU 486.

REFERENCES

1. CHANG, M. C. 1950. Development and fate of transferred rabbit ova or blastocyst in relation to the ovulation time of recipients. J. Exp. Zool. **114:** 197-225.
2. PSYCHOYOS, A. 1973. Endocrine control of egg-implantation. *In* Handbook of Physiology, Endocrinology. O. Greep & E. B. Astwood, Eds. **2:** 187-215. Am. Physiological Society. Washington, D.C.
3. NOYES, R. W., Z. DICKMANN & A. H. GATES. 1963. Ovum transfers, synchronous and asynchronous, in the study of implantation. *In* Delayed Implantation. A. C. Enders, Ed.: 197-211. University of Chicago Press.
4. MCLAREN, A. & D. MICHIE. 1956. Studies on the transfer of fertilized mouse eggs to uterine foster-mothers. I. Factors affecting the implantation and survival of native and transferred eggs. J. Exp. Biol. **33:** 394-416.
5. LAWSON, R. A. S. 1977. *In* Embryo Transfer in Farm animals. K. H. Betteridge, Ed. **16:** 72-78. Agriculture. Canada.
6. PSYCHOYOS, A. & V. CASIMIRI. 1980. Factors involved in uterine receptivity and refractoriness. Prog. Reprod. Biol. **7:** 143-157. Karger. Basel.
7. KENNEDY, T. G. 1979. Prostaglandins and increased endometrial vascular permeability resulting from the application of an artificial stimulus to the uterus of the rat sensitized for the decidual cell reaction. Biol. Reprod. **20:** 560-566.
8. SHELESNYAK, M. C. & G. J. MARCUS. 1969. The study of nidation. *In* Ovum Implantation. M. C. Shelesnyak, Ed.: 3-30. Gordon and Breach. New York.
9. NOYES, R. W., A. T. HERTIG & J. ROCK. 1950. Dating the endometrial biopsy. Fertil. Steril. **1:** 3-25.
10. MARTIN, L. & C. A. FINN. 1968. Hormonal regulation of cell division in epithelial and connective tissues of the mouse uterus. J. Endocrinol. **41:** 363-371.
11. TACHI, C., S. TACHI & H. R. LINDNER. 1972. Modification by progesterone of oestradiol-induced cell proliferation, RNA synthesis and oestradiol distribution in the rat uterus. J. Reprod. Fertil. **31:** 59-76.
12. PSYCHOYOS, A. & P. MANDON. 1971. Etude de la surface de l'épithélium utérin sur

microscope électronique à balayage. Observations chez la ratte au 4è et au 5è jour de la gestation. C. R. Acad. Sci. (Paris) **272:** 2723-2725.

13. ENDERS, A. C. & D. M. NELSON. 1973. Pinocytotic activity in the uterus of the rat. Am. J. Anat. **138:** 277-299.

14. PARR, M. B. & E. L. PARR. 1974. Uterine luminal epithelium protrusions mediate endocytosis, not apocrine secretion in the rat. Biol. Reprod. **11:** 220-223.

15. MARTEL, D., C. MALET, J. P. GAUTRAY & A. PSYCHOYOS. 1981. Surface changes of the luminal uterine epithelium during the human menstrual cycle: a scanning electron microscopic study. *In* The Endometrium: Hormonal Impacts. J. de Brux, R. Mortel & J. P. Gautray, Eds.: 15-29. Plenum Press. New York.

16. ENDERS, A. C. & S. SCHLAFKE. 1974. Surface coats of the mouse blastocyst and uterus during the preimplantation period. Anat. Rec. **180:** 31-46.

17. CHAVEZ, D. J. & T. L. ANDERSON. 1985. The glycocalyx of the mouse uterine luminal epithelium during estrus, early pregnancy, the peri-implantation period and delayed implantation. I. Acquisition of Ricinus communis binding sites during pregnancy. Biol. Reprod. **32:** 1135-1142.

18. MORRIS, J. E. & S. W. POTTER. 1984. A comparison of developmental changes in surface charge in mouse blastocysts and uterine epithelium using DEAE Beads and Dextran sulfate *in vitro.* Dev. Biol. **103:** 190-199.

19. RATH, N. C., C. OLMEDO, V. CASIMIRI, S. PARVEZ, D. ROCHE, H. PARVEZ & A. PSYCHOYOS. 1979. Monoamine metabolism during early pregnancy in the rat. *In* Research on Steroids **8:** 11-15. Academic Press. New York.

20. KREITMANN, O., S. AMR, F. BAYARD & J. C. FAYE. 1980. Measurement of estradiol-17 beta dehydrogenase activity in rat endometrium during the estrous cycle and the first half of pregnancy. Biol. Reprod. **22:** 155-158.

21. PSYCHOYOS, A. 1960. Nouvelle contribution à l'étude de la nidation de l'oeuf chez la ratte. C. R. Acad. Sci. (Paris) **251:** 3073-3075.

22. KRAICER, P. F. & M. C. SHELESNYAK. 1959. Détermination de la période de sensibilité maximale de l'endomètre à la décidualisation au moyen de déciduomes provoqués par un traitement empruntant la voie vasculaire. C. R. Acad. Sci. (Paris) **248:** 3213-3215.

23. DE FEO, V. J. 1963. Determination of the sensitive period for the induction of deciduomata in the rat by different inducing procedures. Endocrinology **73:** 488-497.

24. DICKMANN, Z. & R. W. NOYES. 1960. The fate of ova transferred into the uterus of the rat. J. Reprod. Fertil. **12:** 197-212.

25. PSYCHOYOS, A. 1966. Recent research on egg-implantation. *In* Ciba Foundation Study Group on Egg Implantation. G. E. W. Wolstenholme & M. O'Connor, Eds.: 4-28 Churchill. London.

26. PSYCHOYOS, A. 1976. Hormonal control of uterine receptivity for nidation. J. Reprod. Fertil. Suppl. **25:** 17-28.

27. MARTEL, D. & A. PSYCHOYOS. 1982. Different responses of rat endometrial epithelium and stroma to induction of oestradiol binding sites by progesterone. J. Reprod. Fertil. **64:** 387-389.

28. GLASSER, S. R. & S. A. McCORMACK. 1981. Separated cell types as analytical tools in the study of decidualization and implantation. *In* Cellular and Molecular Aspects of Implantation. S. R. Glasser & D. W. Bullock, Eds.: 217-239. Plenum Press. New York.

29. GLASSER, S. R. & S. A. McCORMACK. 1979. Estrogen modulated uterine gene transcription in relation to decidualization. Endocrinology **104:** 1112-1118.

30. MEYERS, K. 1970. Hormonal requirements for the maintenance of oestradiol-induced inhibition of uterine sensitivity in the ovariectomized rat. J. Endocrinol. **46:** 341-346.

31. PHILIBERT, D., R. DERAEDT, G. TEUTSCH, C. TOURNEMINE & E. SAKIZ. 1982. RU 38486- A new lead for steroidal anti-hormones. Endocrine Society, 64th annual meeting. San Francisco, Abstr. n° 668.

32. WANG, M. Y., V. RIDER, R. B. HEAP & A. FEINSTEIN. 1984. Action of anti-progesterone monoclonal antibody in blocking pregnancy after postcoital administration in mice. J. Endocrinol. **101:** 95-100.

Prostaglandins and Uterine Sensitization for the Decidual Cell Reaction[a]

T. G. KENNEDY

MRC Group in Reproductive Biology
Departments of Obstetrics and Gynaecology, and Physiology
The University of Western Ontario
London, Ontario, Canada N6A 5A5

INTRODUCTION

There are considerable differences among species in the process of implantation, most notably in the extent of trophoblastic invasion of the endometrium.[1,2] In all species, however, embryo-uterine interactions resulting in successful implantation can be initiated only when the embryo and endometrium have reached a precise stage of maturity. The embryo has to be at the blastocyst stage of development, and hormone-dependent changes, leading to the development of a receptive (or sensitized) endometrium, must have occurred. Lack of synchronization in the development of the embryo and endometrium results in the failure, or less commonly, the postponement, of implantation.

In rodents, the regulation of uterine sensitization has most commonly been investigated in pseudopregnant or ovariectomized, hormone-treated animals. In these studies the blastocyst is usually replaced by an artifical stimulus.[3] This situation has an advantage because the stimulus applied to the uterus can be standardized. In response to artificial stimuli, sensitized uteri undergo decidualization, that is, endometrial stromal cells undergo growth and differentiation to decidual cells, giving rise to what would be the maternal component of the placenta during normal pregnancy.[2] Decidualization, whether in response to natural, blastocyst-derived stimuli, or to artificial stimuli, is always preceded by an increase in endometrial vascular permeability.

Studies in rodents have indicated that the uterus will undergo decidualization in response to artificial stimuli for only a limited time during pregnancy, pseudopregnancy, or when the uterus has been prepared by an

[a]The author's research reported in this review was supported by The Medical Research Council of Canada.

appropriate regimen of hormone treatments.[2-4] In addition, uterine sensitization is exquisitely hormone-dependent; estrogens in low dosages act synergistically with progesterone to produce sensitization, at least in the rat and mouse.[2-4] Too high a dose of estrogen results in a nonsensitized uterus.

Mechanisms operating at the cellular level to regulate uterine sensitization are poorly understood. There is now considerable evidence that prostaglandins (PGs) have an important role, likely not acting alone but in concert with other compounds, in mediating both the endometrial vascular changes and the subsequent decidualization (reviewed by Kennedy[5]). It is, therefore, possible that changes in uterine sensitization are related to the ability of the uterus to produce or respond to PGs. Investigations that addressed these possibilities will be reviewed here.

SENSITIZATION AND UTERINE PROSTAGLANDIN PRODUCTION

That changes in uterine sensitization might be related to the ability of the uterus to produce PGs was suggested first by reports that the production of PGs by uterine homogenates from pregnant and pseudopregnant rats is maximal on day 5,[6,7] corresponding to when the uterus is most sensitive to deciduogenic stimuli, and secondly by observation that ovarian steroid hormones affect uterine PG production.[8-10] Investigations, however, of the timing of uterine sensitization and its modification with estrogen,[12] in which uterine PG concentrations after the application of a standardized deciduogenic stimulus were used to assess uterine PG production, indicated that uterine PG levels did not provide a ready explanation for changes in uterine sensitization in the rat. In virtually all cases, the deciduogenic stimulus increased uterine PG concentrations; the magnitude of the increase varied and was not related to uterine sensitization. Milligan and Lytton[13] have made similar observations in the mouse.

It should be noted that these investigations cannot be considered as definitive because uterine PG concentrations were measured in the whole uterus in an attempt to assess uterine PG production. Presumably it is endometrial PG production and endometrial PG concentrations that are relevant for decidualization. Unfortunately, it is at present not technically possible to determine the relative contributions of endometrium and myometrium to the elevated uterine PG concentrations that have been observed after uterine stimulation.

SENSITIZATION AND PROSTAGLANDIN-INDUCED INCREASES IN ENDOMETRIAL VASCULAR PERMEABILITY

As with decidualization, the increase in endometrial vascular permeability in response to an artifical deciduogenic stimulus is time- and hormone-dependent.[11,12] Because assessment of PG production following uterine stimulation did not allow definitive conclusions, it was of interest to determine the ability of sensitized and nonsensitized uteri to respond to exogenously administered PGs. These experiments were performed in rats treated with indomethacin, an inhibitor of PG biosynthesis;[14] in these circumstances, the response obtained is more likely to be due to the exogenous PG, rather than an interaction between the exogenous PG and endogenously produced PGs. Endometrial vascular permeability was chosen as the end point because an increase in permeability is one of the earliest responses of the sensitized uterus to uterine stimulation. The rationale for the experiments was as follows: if lack of uterine sensitization was a consequence of a reduced ability of the uterus to produce PGs, then exogenous PGs should be capable of producing as great an increase in endometrial vascular permeability in the nonsensitized uterus as in the sensitized uterus.

The results obtained indicated that when PGE_2 or its vehicle was injected into the uterine lumen of rats with differentially sensitized uteri, the greatest response in endometrial vascular permeability occurred in the optionally sensitized animals.[11,12] These data suggest that it is the ability of the uterus to respond to PGs that determines, at least in part, uterine sensitization. They also suggest that changes in the ability of the uterus to produce PGs in response to deciduogenic stimuli are of secondary importance in regulating uterine sensitization.

There are several possible explanations for the findings that uterine responsiveness to PGs changes in differentially sensitized uteri. Endometrial responsiveness may be related to the properties of endometrial receptors for PGs that may, for example, be present in the greatest concentrations in the maximally sensitized uterus. Alternatively, changes in endometrial vascular permeability may require mediators in addition to PGs, and it may be the production, release, or action of these compounds that determines maximum uterine sensitization. Finally, the exogenously administered PGs may have been cleared so rapidly from the nonsensitized uteri that they were ineffective. These possibilities have been investigated to a certain extent.

SENSITIZATION AND ENDOMETRIAL PROSTAGLANDIN RECEPTORS

Membrane preparations from sensitized rat endometrium contain specific, saturable, high-affinity PGE-binding sites that may represent PGE receptors. Equivalent binding sites for $PGF_{2\alpha}$ have not been detected.[16]

Whereas the concentrations of PGE-binding sites in the endometrium are time- and hormone-dependent,[15,17] the changes do not provide a ready explanation for changes in uterine sensitization. For example, whereas the increase in the concentration of endometrial binding sites for PGE_2 between days 4 and 5 of pseudopregnancy may possibly explain the onset of uterine responsiveness to PGE, the termination of responsiveness on day 6 cannot be explained in these terms, because PGE_2 binding site concentrations are higher on day 6 than on day five.

PGE binding sites within the endometrium may not always represent "functional" receptors for PGE. This possibility is difficult to address because, at present, the "second messenger" for PGE_2 within the endometrium is uncertain; investigation of cyclic AMP as the second messenger has produced equivocal results.[18] However, because of the ability of exogenously administered PGE to increase uterine cyclic AMP concentrations, it is clear that there are functional PGE_2 receptors in sensitized and nonsensitized uteri.[19,20]

SENSITIZATION AND MEDIATORS IN ADDITION TO PROSTAGLANDINS

The possibility that other mediators acting with PGs may be required to increase endometrial vascular permeability and that it is the production, release, or action of these compounds that determines maximum uterine sensitization has been investigated in part. A major barrier to these investigations is the identity of the putative additional mediator(s). Power and Kennedy[21] were unable to override estrogen-induced unresponsiveness by the intrauterine injection of PGE_2 combined with either histamine or bradykinin. In this study, however, it was not known if histamine or bradykinin were able to reach their presumed site of action, the endothelial cells within the endometrium. There is suggestive evidence of a barrier to the free movement of some compounds out of the uterine lumen into the endometrium.[22]

SENSITIZATION AND UTERINE CLEARANCE OF PROSTAGLANDINS

The nonsensitized uterus may be less responsive to exogenously administered PGs because of rapid clearance of the PGs, either by metabolism or by translocation across the uterine wall. In the rabbit, the rates of translocation of PGs across the uterine wall varies throughout early pregnancy and pseudopregnancy.[23] In rats, the possibility of more rapid clearance from nonsensitized uteri has not been examined directly; an indirect approach, however, has been made.[24] The ability of differentially sensitized uteri to undergo decidualization when exposed to elevated PG levels over an extended time has been investigated; elevated PG levels were achieved by the intrauterine infusion of PGs from Alzet osmotic minipumps.[25,26] The rationale for these experiments was that if clearance of PGs from the nonsensitized uteri was the basis of the reduced response, then the infusion of PGs should result in equivalent decidualization in sensitized and nonsensitized uteri.

The ability of PGs to produce decidualization when infused into nonsensitized uteri varied from no effect to producing almost as much decidualization as in the maximally sensitized animals. The data thus indicated that temporal and hormonal changes in uterine sensitization can at best be partially circumvented by the intrauterine infusion of PGs. Hence it is unlikely that the reduced decidual cell reaction in nonsensitized uteri can be attributed simply to insufficiently elevated levels of endogenously produced PGs following the application of deciduogenic stimuli.

CONCLUSIONS

Mechanisms operating at the cellular level to regulate uterine sensitization for the decidual cell reaction remain poorly understood. Whereas PGs clearly have a role in decidualization, little is known about their site or mechanism of action within the endometrium. Elucidation of these may provide important insights into the control of uterine sensitization because changes in endometrial responsiveness to PGs change in parallel with sensitization.

REFERENCES

1. AMOROSO, E. C. 1952. Placentation. *In* Marshall's Physiology of Reproduction. A. S. Parkes, Ed.: Vol. III: 127-311. Longmans, Green and Co. London.
2. PSYCHOYOS, A. 1973. Endocrine control of egg implantation. *In* Handbook of Physiology. R. O. Greep, E. B. Astwood & S. R. Geiger, Eds.: Section 7, Vol. 2 Part 2: 187-215. American Physiological Society. Bethesda, Md.
3. FINN, C. A. & D. G. PORTER. 1975. The Uterus. Publishing Sciences Group. Acton, Mass.
4. DE FEO, V. J. 1967. Decidualization. *In* Cellular Biology of the Uterus. R. M. Wynn, Ed.: 191-290. Meredith Publishing Co. New York.
5. KENNEDY, T. G. 1983. Embryonic signals and the initiation of blastocyst implantation. Aust. J. Biol. Sci. **36:** 531-543.
6. FENWICK, L., R. L. JONES, B. NAYLOR, N. L. POYSER & N. H. WILSON, 1977. Production of prostaglandins by the pseudopregnant rat uterus, *in vitro,* and the effect of tamoxifen with the identification of 6-keto-prostaglandin $F_{1\alpha}$ as a major product. Br. J. Pharmacol. **59:** 191-199.
7. PHILLIPS, C. A. & N. L. POYSER. 1981. Studies on the involvement of prostaglandins in implantation in the rat. J. Reprod. Fertil. **62:** 73-81.
8. CASTRACANE, V. D. & V. J. JORDAN. 1975. The effect of estrogen and progesterone on uterine prostaglandin biosynthesis in the ovariectomized rat. Biol. Reprod. **13:** 587-596.
9. KUEHL, F. A., V. J. CIRILLO, M. E. ZANETTI, G. C. BEVERIDGE & E. A. HAM. 1976. The effect of estrogen upon cyclic nucleotide and prostaglandin levels in rat uterus. Adv. Prostaglandin Thromboxane Res. **1:** 313-323.
10. PAKRASI, P. L., H. C. CHEUNG & S. K. DEY. 1983. Prostaglandins in the uterus: modulation by steroid hormones. Prostaglandins **26:** 991-1009.
11. KENNEDY, T. G. 1980. Timing of uterine sensitivity for the decidual cell reaction: role of prostaglandins. Biol. Reprod. **22:** 519-525.

12. KENNEDY, T. G. 1980. Estrogen and uterine sensitization for the decidual cell reaction: role of prostaglandins. Biol. Reprod. **23:** 955-962.
13. MILLIGAN, S. R. & F. D. C. LYTTON. 1983. Changes in prostaglandin levels in the sensitized and nonsensitized uterus of the mouse after the intrauterine instillation of oil or saline. J. Reprod. Fertil. **67:** 373-377.
14. VANE, J. R. 1971. Inhibition of prostaglandin synthesis as a mechanism of action of aspirin-like drugs. Nature (London) New Biol. **231:** 232-235.
15. KENNEDY, T. G., D. MARTEL & A. PSYCHOYOS. 1983. Endometrial prostaglandin E_2 binding: characterization in rats sensitized for the decidual cell reaction and changes during pseudopregnancy. Biol. Reprod. **29:** 556-564.
16. MARTEL, D., T. G. KENNEDY, M. N. MONIER & A. PSYCHOYOS. 1985. Failure to detect prostaglandin $F_{2\alpha}$ binding sites in membrane preparations from rat endometrium. J. Reprod. Fertil. **75:** 265-274.
17. KENNEDY, T. G., D. MARTEL & A. PSYCHOYOS. 1983. Endometrial prostaglandin E_2 binding during the estrous cycle and its hormonal control in ovariectomized rats. Biol. Reprod. **29:** 565-571.
18. KENNEDY, T. G. 1983. Prostaglandin E_2, adenosine 3':5'-cyclic monophosphate and changes in endometrial vascular permeability in rat uteri sensitized for the decidual cell reaction. Biol. Reprod. **29:** 1069-1076.
19. JOHNSTON, M. E. A. & T. G. KENNEDY. 1984. Estrogen and uterine sensitization for the decidual cell reaction in the rat: role of prostaglandin E_2 and adenosine 3':5'-cyclic monophosphate. Biol. Reprod. **31:** 959-966.
20. JOHNSTON, M. E. A. & T. G. KENNEDY. 1985. Temporal desensitization of rat uteri for the decidual cell reaction is abolished by cholera toxin acting by a mechanism apparently not involving adenosine 3':5'-cyclic monophosphate. Can. J. Physiol. Pharmacol. **63:** 1052-1056.
21. POWER, S. G. A. & T. G. KENNEDY. 1982. Estrogen induced changes in uterine sensitivity for the decidual cell reaction: interactions between prostaglandin E_2 and histamine or bradykinin. Prostaglandins **23:** 219-226.
22. WALTERS, M. R., R. L. HAZELWOOD & A. L. LAWRENCE. 1979. Amino acid transport from the lumen of the rat uterus. Biol. Reprod. **20:** 985-990.
23. CAO, Z. D., M. A. JONES & M. J. K. HARPER. 1984. Prostaglandin translocation from the lumen of the rabbit uterus *in vitro* in relation to day of pregnancy or pseudopregnancy. Biol. Reprod. **31:** 505-519.
24. KENNEDY, T. G. 1986. Intrauterine infusion of prostaglandins and decidualization in rats with uteri differentially sensitized for the decidual cell reaction. Biol. Reprod. **34:** 327-335.
25. KENNEDY, T. G. & L. A. LUKASH. 1982. Induction of decidualization by the intrauterine infusion of prostaglandins. Biol. Reprod. **27:** 253-260.
26. KENNEDY, T. G. 1985. Evidence for the involvement of prostaglandins throughout the decidual cell reaction in the rat. Biol. Reprod. **33:** 140-146.

Embryonic Signals in Pregnancy[a]

S. K. DEY AND D. C. JOHNSON

Departments of Gynecology and Obstetrics, and Physiology
Ralph L. Smith Research Center
University of Kansas Medical Center
Kansas City, Kansas 66103

The role of estrogen in implantation remains unresolved. In the rat and mouse, this steroid is essential for induction of implantation in the progesterone-primed uterus.[1,2] In other species, such as the rabbit, hamster, or pig, maternal estrogen is not an absolute requirement for implantation.[3-5] In these species either estrogen is not required or it is provided by the implanting blastocyst. Indeed, the ability of the blastocysts of these species to produce estrogen has been demonstrated,[6-10] and there is evidence that estrogen is a requirement for embryo development and implantation.[10-14]

Assuming that under normal conditions estrogen plays an important or essential role in implantation, we can raise questions regarding the mechanisms involved. Increased uterine stromal capillary permeability at the location of the blastocyst is one of the earliest manifestations of implantation.[1] Early studies,[15] particularly those of our honoree, implicated histamine, released from mast cells, as the agent responsible for the permeability changes. The prompt release of histamine in response to estrogen exposure has been demonstrated repeatedly.[16,17] More recent attention has focused upon the vasoactive action of prostaglandins for altering capillary permeability during the implantation process.[18] Estrogen increases prostaglandin synthesis in the progesterone-primed uterus.[19] A complicating factor is that neither histamine release nor prostaglandin synthesis in response to estrogen is altered by the administration of antiestrogen or inhibitors of RNA or protein synthesis.[19,20] These findings contribute to the suggestion that some important functions of estrogen are not mediated by way of the classical cytosolic-nuclear estrogen receptor.

We have recently proposed that certain aspects of estrogen actions in implantation are mediated by way of catechol estrogens, the major metabolites of phenolic estrogens (FIG. 1). For the present discussion we will address four specific questions: Can catechol estrogens replace phenolic estrogen for initiation of implantation? Can these steroids stimulate prostaglandin synthesis in the target tissues? Where are the catechol estrogens formed? and Can estrogens, with impeded catechol-forming capacity, initiate implantation? For

[a]The original research reported was in part supported by NIH Grants HD-12122 and BRSG SO7RRO5373.

a variety of reasons (hormonal requirements, sample size requirements) the answers to these questions cannot be obtained at present using a single species. We have employed rats, rabbits, and pigs in our attempts at providing answers to the above questions.

EFFECT OF CATECHOL ESTROGENS ON IMPLANTATION

The model of delayed implantation, produced by injecting progesterone daily following hypophysectomy on day 3 of pregnancy (day 1 = morning of finding spermatozoa in the vagina) was used to determine the effects of catechol estradiols on implantation in the rat. For reasons not completely understood, these animals are exquisitely sensitive to estradiol for induction

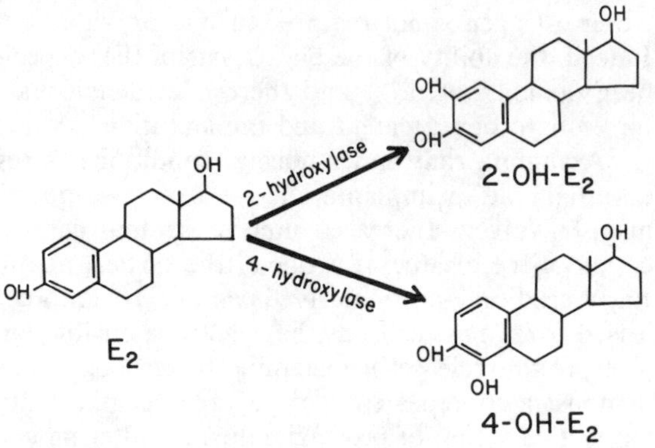

FIGURE 1. The structure of 2-hydroxyestradiol (2-OH-E$_2$) and 4-hydroxyestradiol (4-OH-E$_2$) produced by the action of estrogen-2/4-hydroxylase upon estradiol-17β (E$_2$).

of implantation.[21] The effectiveness of 4-hydroxyestradiol (4-OH-E$_2$) and 2-hydroxyestradiol (2-OH-E$_2$) on induction of implantation in this model was compared to that of estradiol-17β (E$_2$). Because of the rapid degradation and clearance of catechol estradiols, they were administered, either by a single subcutaneous injection, or by way of osmotic minipumps at a constant infusion rate for varying periods. The experimental protocol is shown in FIGURE 2. The animals were checked for implantation sites 24 hours following the installation of pumps or the subcutaneous injection of estrogens. They were injected (i.v.) with 1 ml of a 2% solution of Chicago Blue B in saline, under light ether anesthesia, 15 minutes before killing with an overdose of ether. The presence of blue reaction sites, indicative of increased uterine stromal capillary permeability,[1] was taken as evidence of initiation of implantation. The uteri were flushed with 0.5 ml of saline to confirm the presence of blastocysts. Occasionally, sperm positive animals were without sites or blas-

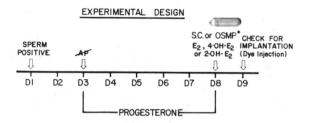

FIGURE 2. Schematic presentation of the protocol used for the hypophysectomized (AP) delayed implanting rat. All animals received 2 mg of progesterone (s.c.) daily prior to estrogen treatment.

tocysts, and they were excluded from the study. As shown in TABLE 1, injection of progesterone in hypophysectomized pregnant rats failed to induce implantation, but subcutaneous injection of 100 ng of E_2 resulted in a normal complement of sites in all of the animals. By contrast, a subcutaneous injection of either 100 or 200 ng of 4-OH-E_2 was quite ineffective in inducing the blue reaction. Increasing the dose to 400 ng/rat, however, resulted in the normal number of implantations in all animals.

TABLE 2 shows the results of infusion of estrogen by osmotic minipumps on implantation. While infusion of the vehicle did not initiate implantation, blue reaction sites were present in all animals infused for 6 or 24 hours with E_2 at the rate of 10 ng/hour. Infusion of 4-OH-E_2 (10 ng/hr) for 24 hours showed no effect on implantation but increasing the rate to 25 or 50 ng/hr induced sites in all animals. Infusion of 4-OH-E_2 at 50 ng/hr for 6 or 8 hours also resulted in implantations in most animals when they were examined 24 hours later. By contrast, 2-OH-E_2 at 50 ng/hr for 24 hours was not effective in initiating implantation. Administering 200 ng/hr for 24 hours, however, initiated implantation in 50% of the rats.

TABLE 1. The Effect of a Single Subcutaneous Injection of Estrogens upon Implantation in the Hypophysectomized Delayed Implanting Rat[a]

Treatment	Dose (ng/rat)	Rats with sites / Number of rats	Number of sites per rat	Number of blastocysts recovered
Oil control	—	0/8	0	9.7 ± 0.3
Estradiol-17β	100	3/3	$8.7 \pm 1.5^{\#}$	5.0 ± 2.3
4-Hydroxyestradiol	100 or 200	2/8	5-6	9.9 ± 0.9
	400	6/6	$8.3 \pm 1.1^{\#}$	5.5 ± 1.4

[a] $\pm$ SEM. All rats were injected (s.c.) with 2 mg of progesterone daily preceding the injection of estrogen. Animals were killed 24 h after injection of estrogen. Means with the same superscript symbol are not statistically (chi square) different ($p > 0.05$). Mean number of blastocysts recovered was not different.

TABLE 2. Effect of Continuous Delivery of Estrogens by way of Osmotic Minipump upon Implantation in the Hypophysectomized Delayed Implanting Rat[a]

Treatment	Group	Dose (ng/h)	Duration (h)	Rats with sites / No. of rats	No. of blue sites	No. of blastocysts recovered
Vehicle	1	—	24	0/4	0^1	8.0 ± 1.5
Estradiol	2	10	24	6/6	10.2 ± 1.4^2	5.3 ± 1.1
	3	10	6	6/6	11.2 ± 1.1^2	5.3 ± 0.7
4-Hydroxy-estradiol	4	10	24	0/7	0^1	8.9 ± 1.4
	5	25	24	5/5	9.2 ± 1.7^2	4.1 ± 1.1
	6	50	24	6/6	10.7 ± 1.8^2	4.7 ± 2.5
	7	50	6	4/6	7.5 ± 1.2^2	6.1 ± 1.3
	8	50	8	5/6	8.2 ± 1.8^2	4.5 ± 1.2
2-Hydroxy-estradiol	9	50	24	0/4	0^1	9.0 ± 1.1
	10	200	24	3/6	5.7 ± 2.6^2	7.7 ± 1.3

[a] $\pm$ SEM. All animals were treated with progesterone (2 mg/day) for the 5 days preceding implantation of the minipumps. Animals were killed 24 h after installation of the pumps. All means with the same superscript are not statistically different (p > 0.05) from each other; only animals with sites are included in the means. Means of the number of blastocysts recovered were not statistically different from each other.[35]

EFFECT OF CATECHOL ESTRADIOLS ON PROSTAGLANDIN SYNTHESIS

Although considerable aromatase activity (formation of estradiol-17β) has been documented for rabbit blastocysts at about the time of implantation, [6-8] its role in embryo development and implantation remains an enigma. One of several possibilities is that the enzyme is important for synthesis of estrogen, that is then converted to catechol estrogen in the target tissue. These catechol estrogens could then stimulate prostaglandin production in the blastocyst and/or the endometrium. The prostaglandins then act to trigger the process of implantation. Therefore, we examined prostaglandin production *in vitro* in response to catechol estrogens using rabbit blastocyst and endometrial cells on day 6 of pregnancy (day 1 = 24 h post coitum). The details of this study have been published.[22]

Day 6 rabbit blastocysts (group of 4-6) were incubated for a total of 8 hours following a one-hour preincubation.[22] Media (RPMI-1640) were changed every two hours and stored at $-80°$ C until the prostaglandins were measured by radioimmunoassay.[22] E_2, 4-OH-E_2, or 2-OH-E_2 were added during the second and fourth periods; the vehicle was added during the first and third periods as shown in FIGURE 3.

Single cell suspensions of endometrial tissues from day 6 of pregnancy were prepared as described previously.[23] The cell suspensions (0.5 ml in RPMI-1640) were incubated for two hours in the presence or absence of various estrogens. The media were separated from the cells by centrifugation at 4° C and stored at −80° C. Prostaglandins in the media and the tissues were measured by radioimmunoassays. Based upon cross-reactivities of the antibodies, the prostaglandins assayed are referred to as prostaglandin F and prostaglandin E-A.

As shown in FIGURE 4a and b, the release of prostaglandins from the blastocysts were stimulated by 4-OH-E$_2$ at a concentration of 44 μM or higher, whereas a lower concentration of 8.8 μM did not show any noticeable effect. Stimulation of release of these prostaglandins was also observed when blastocysts were exposed to 44 μM 2-OH-E$_2$. By contrast, E$_2$, at any concentration, either showed no or inhibitory effects on the release of prostaglandins from the blastocysts. Similarly, prostaglandin production by the endometrial cells was stimulated by 4-OH-E$_2$ or 2-OH-E$_2$ when compared to vehicle-treated or E$_2$-treated cells, and the stimulation was dose-related (FIG. 5a,b).

CATECHOL ESTROGEN-FORMING CAPACITY IN THE BLASTOCYST

Pregnancy recognition and increased uterine vascular permeability at the location of the blastocyst (indicative of initiation of implantation) occur between days 12 and 13 in the pig.[24-26] The mechanism is not clearly understood, but estrogen of blastocyst origin has been implicated as an embryonic signal in implantation. If catechol estrogens are more potent than their phenolic counterparts in stimulating prostaglandin production, one could imagine that the blastocyst exerts uterine vascular effects by conversion of phenolic estro-

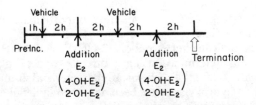

FIGURE 3. The experimental design used to determine the effect of estradiol (E$_2$) and catechol estradiols (2-OH-E$_2$ and 4-OH-E$_2$) on PG synthesis by rabbit day 6 blastocysts. Following a 1 h preincubation period, blastocysts (4-6/group) were alternatively exposed to the steroids or to the vehicle (ethanol:saline mixture, <0.5% ethanol) used to dissolve the steroids. Media were changed at each point indicated with an arrow and saved for assay of protaglandins. After each 2 h incubation period, blastocysts were washed twice with fresh medium at 37° C. (P. L. Pakrasi & S. K. Dey.[22] With permission from *Biology of Reproduction*.)

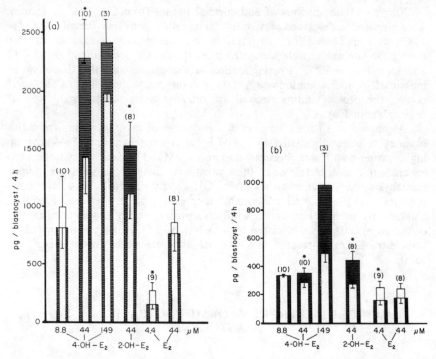

FIGURE 4. The effects of estradiol and catechol estradiols on the release of prostaglandin F **(a)** and prostaglandin E-A**(b)** by day 6 rabbit blastocysts *in vitro.* Vehicle (open bar): first and third incubations. Steroids (solid bar): second and fourth incubations. Statistical analyses were performed by using a two-tailed matched-paired *t* test. The number of experiments is shown in parentheses. Results shown are mean ± SEM; differences in means with p values less than 0.05 were considered significant (*). (P. L. Pakrasi & S. K. Dey.[22] With permission from *Biology of Reproduction.*)

gens to catechol estrogens, which subsequently participate in the local generation of prostaglandins.

Formation of the catechol estradiols, 2-OH-E_2 and 4-OH-E_2 from E_2 by pig blastocysts was determined using a direct product isolation assay for estrogen-2/4-hydroxylase.[27] Biochemical characterization and the temporal pattern of the 2/4-hydroxylase have been described in detail elsewhere.[28] The pattern of the hydroxylase activity in the pig blastocyst on days 10-14 of pregnancy is shown in FIGURE 6. A surge in activity was noticed on days 12 and 13 and was similar to the pattern of aromatase activity (FIG. 7). The activity was limited to extra embryonic tissues. The increases in activity of the estrogen-2/4-hydroxylase and aromatase on days 12 and 13 correlate with the maternal recognition of pregnancy as well as increased uterine blood flow and capillary permeability on these days.[24-26]

EFFECT OF AN ESTROGEN WITH IMPEDED CATECHOL-
FORMING CAPACITY ON IMPLANTATION

More convincing evidence regarding the role of catechol estrogens could be accomplished by use of specific and potent inhibitors of estrogen-2/4-hydroxylase or by use of estrogens with impeded catechol-forming capacity. The former are not available, but fluorinated estradiols are useful for the latter approach. 2-Fluoroestradiol (2-Fl-E_2) and 4-fluoroestradiol (4-Fl-E_2) are relatively potent estrogens in terms of classical cytosolic-nuclear receptor binding, uterotropic effects, and other estrogenic responses,[29-31] but they are poorer substrates than E_2 for catechol estrogen formation.[31] Therefore, we have studied the ability of these fluorinated estradiols to initiate implantation in the rat.

For comparing the implantation-inducing capacity of the fluorinated estradiols with E_2, the hypophysectomized delayed implantation model was used (FIG. 1). On the fifth day of progesterone treatment (day 8 of pregnancy), rats were injected (i.v.) either with saline, 25 ng of E_2, or various amounts of 2-Fl-E_2 or 4-Fl-E_2 dissolved in saline, and killed 24 hours later. Because histamine potentiates the effect of suboptimal doses of E_2 in inducing im-

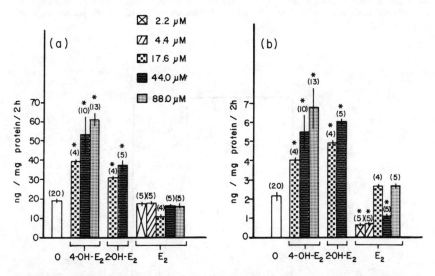

FIGURE 5. The effects of estradiol and catechol estradiols on the production of prostaglandin F (a) and prostaglandin E-A (b) by day 6 rabbit endometrial cells *in vitro*. O = vehicle. Details about the vehicle the same as for FIGURE 3. Bars represent various concentrations of steroids. The production of prostaglandins by the endometrial cells (media plus the cells) is expressed as mean ± SEM. Statistical analyses were performed by one-way analysis of variance and Duncan's multiple range tests. Differences in means with p values less than 0.05 were considered significant. Asterisks denote a significant difference from prostaglandin values in the absence of steroids. The number of experiments is shown in parentheses. (P. L. Pakrasi & S. K. Dey.[22] With permission from *Biology of Reproduction*.)

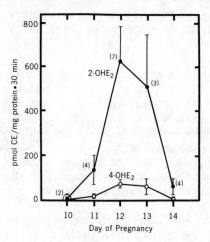

FIGURE 6. Estrogen-2/4-hydroxylase activity in pig blastocysts. Aliquots of blastocyst homogenate were assayed for E-2/4-H. The tritiated catechol estrogens (CE), 2- and 4-hydroxyestradiol (2- and 4-OH-E_2) were isolated by adsorption to neutral alumina and separated by thin layer chromatography. Formation of 2- and 4-OH-E_2 is expressed as picomoles CE/mg protein for 30 minutes. Day of pregnancy is indicated on the horizontal axis. Blastocysts from each pig were pooled and assayed separately. The numbers of pools of blastocysts are indicated in parentheses. Each point is the mean ± SE. (J. S. Mondschein *et al.*[28] With permission from *Endocrinology.*)

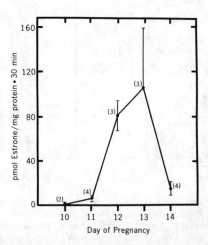

FIGURE 7. Aromatase activity in pig blastocysts. Aliquots of blastocyst homogenate from samples assayed for estrogen-2/4-hydroxylase were also assayed the same day for aromatase activity as described. Aromatase activity is expressed as pmoles estrone/mg protein for 30 minutes. The numbers of pools of blastocysts are indicated in parentheses. Each point is the mean ± SE. (J. S. Mondschein *et al.*[28] With permission from *Endocrinology.*)

plantation in our model, [21] the effects of coadministration of this amine with
2-Fl-E_2 on implantation were also determined. The animals were injected
(i.p.) on day 8 with histamine dihydrochloride (300 μmole/kg) followed 10
minutes later by a single i.v. injection of 30, 75, or 150 ng of 2-Fl-E_2. They
were given two additional i.p. injections of histamine 4 hours apart on the
same day and killed 24 hours after the initial injection.

In order to demonstrate that 2-Fl-E_2 did not have toxic effects upon the
embryo, delayed implanting rats were infused (s.c.) with 4-OH-E_2 (50 ng/
hr) by way of osmotic minipump for 24 hours immediately after injection of
150 ng of 2-Fl-E_2 on day 8 of pregnancy. Rats were killed 24 hours after
injection and initiation of implantation determined by injection (i.v.) of Chicago Blue B as described earlier. As shown in TABLE 2 this dosage of catechol
estradiol when given alone induced implantation in all animals.

To compare the uterotropic effects of 2-Fl-E_2 with those of E_2 in animals

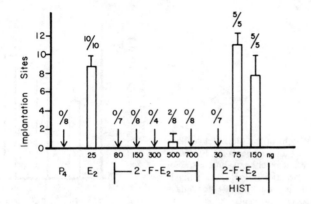

FIGURE 8. The effect of 2-fluoroestradiol (2-F-E_2) upon implantation in the hypophysectomized
delayed implanting rat. All animals received 2 mg of progesterone (P4) daily. The number with
implantation sites/the total number of rats is indicated for each dose. Animals treated with
histamine (HIST) received 300 μmole/kg before as well as four and eight hours after the i.v.
injection of 2-F-E_2.

that do not have the complicating factor of implanting embryos, adult female
rats were hypophysectomized without regard to the stage of the estrous cycle.
Seven days later, the animals were treated (s.c.) with 2 mg of progesterone
daily for 4 days and then given (i.v.) saline, 30 ng of E_2 or 150 ng of 2-Fl-
E_2 dissolved in saline. The animals were killed 24 hours later and their uterine
weights determined.

As shown in FIGURE 8, progesterone treatment alone had no effect, but
superimposition of 25 ng of E_2 promptly initiated implantation in all animals.
By contrast, 2-Fl-E_2 even at the highest dose (700 ng/rat) failed to initiate
implantation; only single sites were noted in 2 of 8 rats injected with 500 ng
of the steroid. The coadministration of 4-OH-E_2 with 150 ng of 2-Fl-E_2
resulted in a full complement of implantation sites (10.9.9 $\pm$ 0.8, N=7) in
all animals. 4-Fl-E_2 was more effective than 2-Fl-E_2, but somewhat less ef-

fective than E_2 at initiating implantation. Whereas a single injection of 30 ng of 4-Fl-E_2 produced sites in 57% of the animals, increasing the dose to 60 ng initiated implantation in all animals. As shown in FIGURE 9, increase in uterine wet weight (mg/100 g body weight, N=5) in hypophysectomized progesterone-treated nonpregnant rats was comparable after an injection of 30 ng of E_2 or 150 ng of 2-Fl-E_2.

Most interestingly, the coadministration of histamine with the 2-Fl-E_2 was quite effective for induction of implantation. In our previous studies,[21] histamine alone never induced implantation in this model, and as shown in FIGURE 8 when given with 30 ng of 2-Fl-E_2, it was also ineffective. When given with 75 ng of 2-Fl-E_2, however, the normal number of sites were found; increasing the dose to 150 ng/rat did not increase the rate of implantation.

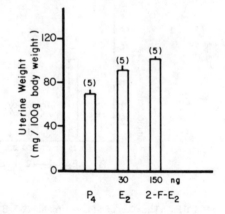

FIGURE 9. Weight of the uteri of hypophysectomized rats (not pregnant) 24 h after a single i.v. injection of either saline, estradiol (E_2), or 2-fluorestradiol (2-F-E_2). All animals received 2 mg of progesterone (P4) for 5 days before the estrogen treatment.

DISCUSSION

We posed four questions, the answers to which could contribute to an understanding of the role of estrogen in implantation. Now the problem is combining the answers we received into a working hypothesis. The expression of estrogenic action in the uterus has been proposed to be mediated by two separate mechanisms, genomic and nongenomic.[32,33] The rapid early responses such as eosinophilia, histamine release, increased prostaglandin synthesis, water imbibition, and vascular reactions are considered to be mediated by way of nongenomic mechanisms. On the other hand, the delayed responses, such as increased RNA, DNA, and protein syntheses are controlled at the genomic level. Unfortunately, we do not know the degree to which these two mechanisms are involved in the process of implantation. The evidence, albeit circumstantial, suggests that both are necessary.

2-Fl-E_2, a relatively potent estrogen in terms of uterotropic (*i.e.* genomic) action, failed to induce implantation even at doses 28 times the effective dose for estradiol. When coadministered with histamine, however, 2-Fl-E_2 induced implantation at a dose only three times that required for estradiol. We interpret this to mean that histamine provided the vasoactive component, whereas 2-Fl-E_2 was responsible for the necessary genomic actions. We further postulate that 2-Fl-E_2 is incapable of providing the nongenomic action of estrogen because it is a poor substrate for estrogen-2/4-hydroxylase[31] and therefore forms a subthreshold amount of catechol estrogen.

If catechol estrogens have an important role in implantation, then they should be able to initiate the process when administered to the delayed implanting animal. Our studies with ovariectomized mice and hypophysectomized rats[34,35] indicate that they have this capability. Estradiol is about 5 times and 20 times more potent than 4-OH-E_2 and 2-OH-E_2, respectively, in inducing implantation in hypophysectomized progesterone-treated delayed implanting rats.[35] This efficacy appears related to the clearance rate of these steroids; the ratio has been reported to be 1:4:11 for E_2, 4-OH-E_2, and 2-OH-E_2.[36] This rapid rate of clearance makes the catechol estrogens poor candidates for circulating hormones. This would be of little consequence, however, if the catechol formation took place in the blastocyst and/or in the endometrium at the location of the blastocyst during the periimplantation period. Thus far, synthesis of the catechol estrogens has been established for the hamster[9] and pig[28] blastocyst, but a recent preliminary report indicated the presence of estrogen-2/4-hydroxylase activity in mouse blastocysts as well.[37] Importantly, the peak in catechol estrogen-forming capacity in the pig blastocyst coincides with several critical events associated with establishment of pregnancy.[24-26]

Why would catechol estrogens be of importance in the implantation process? We believe that their ability to act on more than one receptor system is a key factor. Although the introduction of the second hydroxyl group in the A-ring of estrogens reduces the binding affinity to the cytosolic-nuclear receptor, catechol estrogens can produce the genomic actions of estrogen.[38] Further, because of their structural similarity to the catecholamines, they may be able to function in implantation through blastocyst and endothelial cell membrane interactions.[39] We have demonstrated that they are more potent than phenolic estrogen at inducing synthesis of prostaglandins,[22,40] which are known vasoactive agents associated with the initiation of implantation.[18,21] One must remember that increased prostaglandin synthesis following *in vivo* exposure to estrogen is not altered by antiestrogen, RNA, DNA, or protein synthesis inhibitors.[19]

To synthesize our working hypothesis we have attempted to schematically present the embryo-uterine interactions that bring about vascular permeability changes at the site of implantation (FIGURE 10). Dotted lines indicate questionable or untested pathways. Both phenolic and catechol estrogens can act by way of the genome, but the role of consequent translation products alone in the early phases of implantation may not be adequate. Histamine, released from mast cells in response to estrogen stimulation or produced by the embryo is likely to increase prostaglandin synthesis by stimulating phospholipase A2 action on phospholipids in uterine and embryonic tissues. The effect of catechol estrogen upon histamine release is unknown, but these steroids are vasoactive[41] and are capable of stimulating prostaglandin synthesis. This scheme does not reduce the importance of various hypotheses put forward over the years, but attempts to put them into a comprehensive picture with a new approach to the problem.

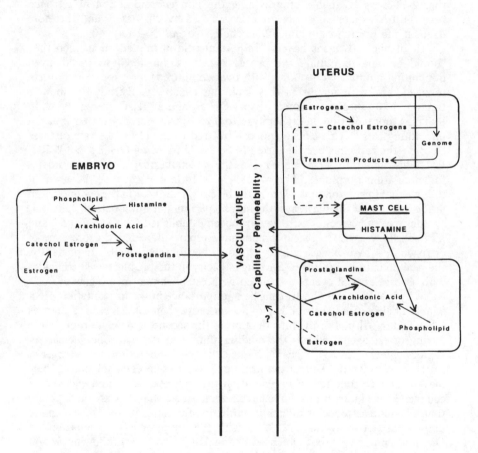

FIGURE 10. Schematic of a working hypothesis for implantation (see text for explanation).

REFERENCES

1. PSYCHOYOS, A. 1974. Hormonal control of ovo-implantation. Vitam. Horm. (NY) **32:** 201-256.
2. YOSHINAGA, K. & C. E. ADAMS. 1966. Delayed implantation in the spayed, progesterone-treated adult mouse. J. Reprod. Fertil. **12:** 593-595.

3. KWUN, J. K. & C. W. EMMENS. 1974. Hormonal requirements for implantation and pregnancy in the ovariectomized rabbit. Aust. J. Biol. Sci. **27:** 275-283.
4. ORSINI, M. W. & R. K. MEYER. 1962. Effect of varying doses of progesterone on implantation in the ovariectomized hamster. Proc. Soc. Exp. Biol. Med. **110:** 713-715.
5. HEAP, R. B., A. P. F. FLINT & J. E. GADSBY. 1981. Embryonic signals and maternal recognition. *In* Cellular and Molecular Aspects of Implantation. S. R. Glasser & D. W. Bullock, Eds.: 311-326. Plenum Press. New York.
6. HOVERSLAND, R. C., S. K. DEY & D. C. JOHNSON. 1982. Aromatase activity in the rabbit blastocyst. J. Reprod. Fertil. **66:** 259-263.
7. GEORGE, F. W. & J. D. WILSON. 1978. Estrogen formation in the early rabbit embryo. Science **199:** 200-201.
8. WU, J. T. & G. M. LIN. 1982. Effect of aromatase inhibitor on oestrogen production in rabbit blastocysts. J. Reprod. Fertil. **66:** 655-662.
9. SHOLL, S. A., M. W. ORSINI & D. J. HITCHINS. 1983. Estrogen synthesis and metabolism in the hamster blastocyst, uterus and liver near the time of implantation. J. Steroid Biochem. **19:** 1153-1161.
10. PERRY, J. S., R. B. HEAP, R. D. BURTON & J. E. GADSBY. 1976. Endocrinology of the blastocyst and its role in the establishment of pregnancy. J. Reprod. Fertil. **25:** (Suppl.) 85-104.
11. PARIA, B. C., J. SENGUPTA & S. K. MANCHANDA. 1984. Role of embryonic oestrogen in rabbit blastocyst development and metabolism. J. Reprod. Fertil. **70:** 429-436.
12. SENGUPTA, J., B. C. PARIA & S. K. MANCHANDA. 1983. Effect of an estrogen antagonist on development of blastocyst and implantation in the hamster. J. Exp. Zool. **225:** 119-122.
13. DEY, S. K., Z. DICKMANN & J. SENGUPTA. 1976. Evidence that the maintenance of early pregnancy in the rabbit requires "blastocyst estrogen." Steroids **28:** 481-485.
14. BHATT, B. M. & D. W. BULLOCK. 1974. Binding of oestradiol to rabbit blastocysts and its possible role in implantation. J. Reprod. Fertil. **39:** 65-70.
15. SHELESNYAK, M. C. 1957. Some experimental studies on the mechanism of ova-implantation in the rat. Recent Prog. Horm. Res. **13:** 269-322.
16. SPAZIANI, E. & C. M. SZEGO. 1958. The influence of estradiol and cortisol on the uterine histamine of the ovariectomized rat. Endocrinology **63:** 669-678.
17. SPAZIANI, E. & C. M. SZEGO. 1959. Further evidence for mediation by histamine of estrogenic stimulation of the uterus. Endocrinology **64:** 713-723.
18. KENNEDY, T. G. 1977. Evidence for a role for prostaglandins in the initiation of blastocyst implantation in the rat. Biol. Reprod. **16:** 286-291.
19. CASTRACANE, V. D. & V. C. JORDAN. 1976. Considerations into the mechanism of estrogen-stimulated uterine prostaglandin synthesis. Prostaglandins **12:** 243-251.
20. MARCUS, G. J. & M. C. SHELESNYAK. 1967. Studies on the mechanism of nidation. XX. Relation of histamine release to estrogen action in the progestational rat. Endocrinology **80:** 1028-1031.
21. JOHNSON, D. C. & S. K. DEY. 1980. Role of histamine in implantation: dexamethasone inhibits estradiol-induced implantation in the rat. Biol. Reprod. **22:** 1136-1141.
22. PAKRASI, P. L. & S. K. DEY. 1983. Catechol estrogens stimulate synthesis of prostaglandins in the preimplantation rabbit blastocysts and endometrium. Biol. Reprod. **29:** 347-354.
23. DEY, S. K., C. VILLANUEVA & N. I. ABDOU. 1979. Histamine receptors on rabbit blastocysts and endometrial cell membranes. Nature (London) **278:** 648-649.
24. DHINDSA, D. S. & P. J. DZIUK. 1968. Effect on pregnancy of killing embryos or fetuses in one uterine horn in early gestation. J. Anim. Sci. **27:** 122-126.
25. FORD, S. P. & R. K. CHRISTENSON. 1979. Blood flow to uteri of sows during the estrous cycle and early pregnancy: Local effect of the conceptus on the uterine blood supply. Biol. Reprod. **21:** 617-624.
26. KEYS, J. L. & G. J. KING. 1985. Changes in vascular permeability and endometrial structure during early gestation in the pig. Biol. Reprod. (Suppl. 1) Abstract 51.
27. HERSEY, R. M., K. I. H. WILLIAMS & J. WEISZ. 1981. Catechol estrogen formation by brain tissue: characterization of a direct product isolation assay for estrogen-2 and 4-hydroxylase activity and its application to studies of 2-and 4-hydroxyestradiol formation by rabbit hypothalamus. Endocrinology **109:** 1912-1920.

28. MONDSCHEIN, J. S., R. M. HERSEY, S. K. DEY, D. L. DAVIS & J. WEISZ. 1985. Catechol estrogen formation by pig blastocysts during the preimplantation period: Biochemical characterization of estrogen-2/4-hydroxylase and correlation with aromatase activity. Endocrinology. **117:** 2339-2346.

29. KATZENELLENBOGEN, J. A., K. E. CARLSON, D. F. HEIMAN & J. E. LLOYD. 1980. Receptor binding as a basis for radiopharmaceutical design. *In* Structure activity relationship. R. E. Spencer, Eds.: 23-86. Grune and Stratton. New York.

30. LIEHR, J. 1983. 2-Fluoroestradiol: Separation of estrogenicity from carcinogenicity. Mol. Pharmacol. **23:** 278-281.

31. KREY, L. C., N. J. MACLUSKY, D. G. PFEIFFER, B. PARSONS, G. R. MERRIAM & F. NAFTOLIN. 1980. *In* Catechol Estrogens. G. R. Merriam & M.B. Lipsett. Eds.: 249-263. Raven Press. New York.

32. TCHERNITCHIN, A. N. 1983. Eosinophil-mediated non-genomic parameters of estrogen stimulation: a separate group of responses mediated by an independent mechanism. J. Steroid Biochem. **19:** 95-100.

33. JENSEN, E. V. & E. R. DESOMBRE. 1972. Mechanism of action of the female sex hormones. Annu. Rev. Biochem. **41:** 203-230.

34. HOVERSLAND, R. C., S. K. DEY & D. C. JOHNSON. 1982. Catechol estradiol induced implantation in the mouse. Life Sci. **30:** 1801-1804.

35. KANTOR, B. S., S. K. DEY & D. C. JOHNSON. 1985. Catechol oestrogen induced initiation of implantation in the delayed implanting rat. Acta Endocrinol. (Copenhagen) **109:** 418-422.

36. BALL, P., G. EMONS, H. KAYSER & J. TEICHMANN. 1983. Metabolic clearance rates of catechol estrogens in rats. Endocrinology **113:** 1781-1783.

37. HOVERSLAND, R. C. 1985. Presence of 2/4-estradiol hydroxylase in mouse embryos collected on day 5 of pregnancy. Biol. Reprod. (Suppl. 1) Abst. 205.

38. HERSEY, R. M., J. WEISZ & B. S. KATZENELLENBOGEN. 1982. Estrogenic potency, receptor interactions and metabolism of catechol estrogens in the immature rat uterus *in vitro.* Endocrinology **111:** 896-903.

39. SCHAEFFER, J., S. STEVENS, R. SMITH & A. HSUEH. 1980. Binding of 2-hydroxyestradiol to rat anterior pituitary cell membranes. J. Biol. Chem. **255:** 9838-9843.

40. KELLY, R. W. & M. H. ABEL. 1981. A comparison of the effects of 4-catechol oestrogens and 2-pyrogallol oestrogens on prostaglandin synthesis by the rat and human uterus. J. Steroid Biochem. **14:** 787-791.

41. STICE, S. L., D. E. VANORDEN & S. P. FORD. 1985. Role of estrogen(E) and catechol estrogen(CE) in reducing uterine arterial tone and 45Ca uptake. Program of Annual Meeting of the Society for Gynecologic Investigation. Abst. 197P.

Tentative Extrapolation of Animal Data to Human Implantation

B. LEJEUNE,[a] M. F. DEHOU,[b] AND F. LEROY[a]

[a]Human Reproduction Research Unit
[b]Department of Pathology
Hôpital Saint Pierre
Free University of Brussels
Brussels, Belgium

INTRODUCTION

For all aspects of implantation, information can be obtained from animal models to help elucidate the processes taking place in our own species. Although extrapolation from one species to another is not easy, animal models are needed for ethical reasons because it is difficult to explore human implantation directly. Furthermore, the timing of implantation in women is less precise. Whereas women may have intercourse at any stage of the cycle, nonhuman species almost always copulate at the appropriate time for successful fertilization and implantation. Finally, because implantation is a recent occurrence in biological evolution, it displays wide interspecies diversity that brings the human closer to some rodents than even to some primates studied so far.

SYNCHRONISM AND THE IMPLANTATION WINDOW

The central theme that emerged from experimental studies on implantation is the necessity of synchronism between embryo and endometrium for successful implantation. This dynamic concept mainly rests on classical transfer experiments carried out on laboratory rodents as well as on large domestic animals. These investigations confirm that endometrial conditions for implantation are rather stringently defined but that a relative behavioral flexibility of the conceptus allows some degree of adaptation to asynchronous conditions.

It is well-known that in rats and mice, synchronous transfer is successful and that embryos older than the recipient uterus will also easily attach.[1] Introduction of embryos, however, into uteri one day older results in failure.

In the mare, transfer of embryos into uteri one day younger seems to entail better results than transfer under strictly synchronous conditions.[2] This property of the embryo to block its development is probably related to the capacity displayed by numerous species to undergo delayed implantation.

A reverse adaptive behavior of the egg has also been reported. Transfer of day 4 sheep embryos to advanced day 7 uteri results in accelerated embryonic growth as compared to the development of synchronously transferred controls.[3] Such transfers to advanced uteri, however, do not lead to evolutive pregnancies.

In rats and mice, uterine receptivity to the embryo is well-defined and short-lived, lasting less than 24 hours. Outside this period, the endometrium is at best indifferent or has become hostile.

The human embryo normally enters the uterine cavity around day 5 after ovulation and attaches soon thereafter. In *in vitro* fertilization (IVF) programs, however, embryos are replaced in the uterus at 45 hr after oocyte retrieval and remain unimplanted for at least four days.

Data recently presented by Lenton[4] on the initiation of human chorionic gonadotropin (hCG) secretion suggest that in the human, endometrial receptivity to implantation may extend from day 5 to day 11 after the luteinizing hormone (LH) surge. It would appear, however, that for successful evolutive pregnancies to occur there is a relatively narrow implantation window of only three days (five to seven). Outside these latter limits implantation often leads to miscarriage.

It has been observed that hCG becomes detectable two days later in IVF pregnancies as compared to pregnancies obtained by artificial insemination or occurring *in vivo* after Clomid/hCG stimulation.[5]

This study was possible because in all these cases the time of ovulation could be precisely determined. Taken together with Lenton's data,[4] these results might explain the higher abortion rate that is observed in all IVF programs. These data also suggest that the human endometrium does not undergo a sharply delineated sequence of events involving neutrality, receptivity, and refractoriness towards the embryo, such as observed in laboratory rodents.

ROLES OF LUTEAL ESTROGEN AND PROGESTERONE

In rats and mice, blastocysts can implant only after the rise of luteal estrogen secretion occurring around day 4 of gestation.[6] Without this nidatory estrogen, eggs will be maintained in a state of metabolic quiescence as long as enough progesterone is available.[7]

Two explanations for the nidatory role of luteal estrogen have been proposed: 1) stimulation of the endometrial synthesis of specific factors that induce blastocyst activation and attachment, and 2) inhibition of the synthesis of intrauterine substances that prevent implantation. Supporting the first hypothesis are the increased uterine RNA and general protein synthesis occurring on day 5,[8] the induction of implantation by uterine RNA extracts,[9,10] and the secretion into the uterine lumen of specific proteins on day 5.[11] On the other hand, a mechanism of action through release from inhibition may be invoked: the reawakening of diapausal embryos after their transplantation to extrauterine sites,[12] the possibility of triggering implantation by giving actinomycin D,[13–15] and the inhibitory influence on blastocysts of uterine flushings from delayed implanting uteri.[16,17] Some of our recent work[18] aims at analyzing this apparent contradiction. Through separation by two-dimensional gel electrophoresis performed after labeling with [^{35}S]methionine, we were able to study the changes in protein synthesis occurring in rat endometrial tissues at the successive hormonal stages leading to implantation (TABLE 1).

The overall effect of progesterone is to switch endometrial protein synthesis from estrogen-dependent low molecular weights to the production of bigger polypeptides.

When the full progestational sequence is given, the final small dose of estradiol (luteal or nidatory estrogen) inhibited the synthesis of all but four of the progesterone-induced polypeptides in the epithelium. Such changes would support the theory that implantation is consecutive to the disappearance of intrauterine inhibitory factors. Four proteins synthesized in the progesterone-dominated epithelium remain present after nidatory estrogen action. This observation is compatible with the hypothesis that implantation is related to intrauterine release of embryotrophic substances. On the other hand, five peptides induced by priming with estradiol, but disappearing under additional progesterone treatment, are again synthesized after giving nidatory estradiol. This latter finding agrees with results showing that implantation of delayed blastocysts can be obtained by intraparametrial injection of uterine RNA extracts from estrogen-treated castrated rats.[10] By contrast, very few modifications were observed in the stroma. Nearly all appearing and disappearing polypeptides are observed in the uterine epithelium after nidatory estrogen administration. This lends support to the theory that luteal estrogen triggers implantation by mainly acting at the level of the uterine epithelium.[19,20] On the whole, our data are compatible with a mechanism involving both lifting of intrauterine inhibition and stimulation by embryotrophic substances.

In rats and mice, luteal estrogen, after providing a favorable uterine environment for implantation for 12 to 18 hours, is also responsible for a refractory state in which the uterus becomes hostile to unimplanted eggs and is no longer capable of decidualizing.[21]

Both the receptive and the refractory state are the successive parts of a biphasic phenomenon induced by small amounts of estrogen on the progesterone-dominated uterus. Some of our earlier work shows that the occurrence of the refractory state also involves protein synthesis, because cycloheximide given before nidatory estrogen proved able to maintain the uterus in its initial neutral state.[22] The basic murine model for implantation differs in several aspects from what happens in many other species.

In animal models, luteal estrogen thus triggers implantation by modulating

TABLE 1. Effects of Progestational Hormones on Rat Endometrial Protein Synthesis (double-dimension electrophoresis)[a]

Polypeptide No.	Molecular Weight (× 10^{-3})	Isoelectric point	Group 2 (E E) Total endometrium	Group 3 (E E -- P P P) Epithelium	Group 3 (E E -- P P P) Stroma	Group 4 (E E -- P P Pe) Epithelium	Group 4 (E E -- P P Pe) Stroma
1	22	5.67				0	0
2	29	6.22	+	-	-	+	+
3	30	5.40	+			+	0
4	36	6.62	+	0	0	0	0
5	37	6.62	+			+	0
6	37	6.37	+	0	0	0	0
7	43	5.88	+			0	0
8	43	5.76	+	-	-	0	0
9	44	6.00	+	-	-	+	0
10	52	6.33	+	-	-	0	0
11	55	6.14	+	-	-	0	0
12	55	6.28	+	-	-	+	0
13	23	5.55		+	+	-	0
14	30	5.50		+	+	0	0
15	32	6.14		+	+	0	0
16	35	5.48		+	0	-	0
17	49	6.20		+	+	-	0
18	53	5.86		+	0	-	0
19	54	5.44		+	0	-	+
20	55	5.86		+	+	-	-
21	72	6.10		+	0	0	0
22	75	6.10		+	+	0	0
23	80	6.24		+	0	-	0
24	80	6.24		+	0	-	0
25	90	5.80		+	0	-	0
26	105	5.78		+	0	-	0

[a] For easy comparison, polypeptides are classified by increasing molecular weight in two successive series (1-12 and 13-26). + = newly appearing or markedly increased synthesis; - = disappearing or markedly reduced synthesis; 0 = not modified by comparison with previous treatment group; control group 1 not indicated. Daily treatments: E = proestrus estradiol (1 µg); - = day of rest; P = progesterone (5 mg); e = nidatory estradiol (50 ng).

in particular the protein content[18] and the pyridine nucleotide content[23] of the uterus, thereby imposing stringent temporal requirements upon the embryonic-endometrial interplay. In many species, including most monkeys, no rise of estrogen occurs during the luteal phase. In the human, a moderate hump of estradiol output is observed after ovulation, but it is doubtful that this secretion triggers implantation as it does in rats and mice.[24] There is, however, indication that human implantation might be related to a critical ratio of estrogen to progesterone secretion in the early luteal phase. In rats and mice, the dose of estradiol efficient for inducing implantation of diapausal blastocysts has a clear-cut upper limit above which the uterus quickly becomes resistant without even going through the receptive state.[21]

In human IVF, in comparing the stimulated cycles leading to clinical pregnancies to those leading to chemical pregnancies and failures, we observe that estradiol tends to fall lower in clinical pregnancies on day 1 of the luteal phase and to remain so until day 8. These results might be interpreted as indicating an unfavorable influence of high levels of estradiol on the implantation process. By contrast, progesterone levels are higher at the first day of the luteal phase of conception versus nonconception cycles. Such a difference had already been shown by Lenton[25] in spontaneous cycles. It is interesting that progesterone levels were significantly lower in our chemical pregnancies. High progesterone levels at the beginning of the luteal phase might thus have a beneficial influence on implantation. Patterns of estradiol and progesterone secretions may also be combined into the ratios between these two hormones (E_2/P). These latter patterns indicate that on the first three days of the luteal phase the difference between clinical and either failures or chemical pregnancies is again significant, low E_2/P ratios resulting more often in evolutive pregnancies. It should be added that E_2/P ratios in spontaneous cycles were found similar to those observed in IVF conception cycles but were significantly lower than in IVF failures.

By plotting the stage of development of embryos at replacement according to the E_2/P ratio of their recipient mother on day 3 of the luteal phase, and considering the outcome of the IVF trial, it was observed that 1) most clinical pregnancies were obtained when the E_2/P ratio was lower than 0.05, 2) a subgroup of chemical pregnancies was related to E_2/P values around 0.055, and 3) only failures were found for higher E_2/P ratio (FIG. 1).

These very early characteristics of the luteal phase in conception cycles, that is, high progesterone levels and low E_2/P ratio, are probably not related to luteotrophic signals originating from the embryos, which, in our IVF program, are replaced in the afternoon of day 2 of the luteal phase. They probably depend on the intrinsic potentialities of the corpus luteum and may be a consequence of the quality of the follicular phase. A positive correlation was indeed observed between follicular estradiol and luteal progesterone in our material. Although it has been experimentally demonstrated in monkeys[26] and in women[27,28] that administration of estradiol can have a luteolytic action, the high luteal estradiol observed in our clomiphene-human menopausal gonadotropin (hMG) stimulated cycles did not seem to have induced such effect: no negative correlation was observed between estradiol on day 3-4 and either progesterone on day 8, or luteal phase duration.

Evidence of shortening of the luteal phase, however, has been reported[29] when a high follicular estradiol peak was observed in cycles stimulated by hMG alone. The comparison of trials ending in failure with trials leading to clinical pregnancies, in the same patients who underwent several stimulated cycles for IVF, confirms that pregnancies are obtained in cycles in which 1) the early luteal E_2/P ratio is low, 2) the progesterone level is higher, and in which 3) follicular estradiol is higher.

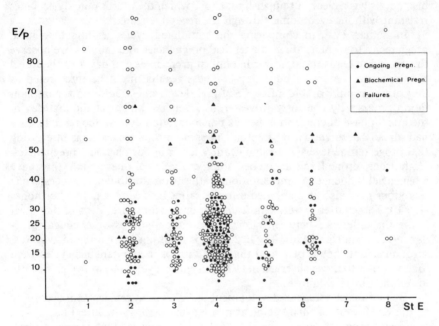

FIGURE 1. Diagram illustrating the endocrine conditions leading to success or failure of implantation in relation to embryonic stage.

MORPHOLOGICAL CORRELATES OF IMPLANTATION

Although morphological criteria are of static nature, they have been the only means so far for directly evaluating human endometrial receptiveness and implantation.

Normally, in the early luteal phase, massive glycogen accumulation is observed around glandular nuclei, and giant mitochrondria surrounded by rough endoplasmic reticulum (RER) are localized at the basal pole of the cell. A basket-like nucleolar channel system appears around day 17, and its maximal development occurs around day 3 after ovulation.[30]

At midluteal phase, the chromatin of the epithelial nuclei is more condensed, secretory activity involving Golgi apparatus and ergastoplasm becomes prominent, and lateral plasma membranes appear more convoluted. More recently, tight junctions have been observed to decrease along the luteal phase.[31] A scanning EM did not show conspicuous changes of the cell surface until day 7 after ovulation.[32]

Few reports dealing with the morphological description of the endometrium in stimulated cycles have been published. Advanced endometrial maturation after ovulation induction with hMG/hCG has been reported.[33] Interestingly, this feature was correlated with higher progesterone levels in the early luteal phase, which is characteristic of conception cycles. In another work,[34] endometrial biopsies were classified as suitable or unsuitable for implantation, and it was concluded that unsuitable endometria were mainly of the underdeveloped type. These patients showed low luteal estradiol and progesterone values, whereas their follicular estradiol peak had also been low.

We were able to investigate 32 endometrial samples: 17 in spontaneous cycles, 11 in clomiphene/hMG/hCG stimulated cycles, and 4 obtained by sequential administration of estradiol with progesterone in premature ovarian failure. Ultrastructural characteristics of the epithelial cells were similar in spontaneous and stimulated cycles. Giant mitochondria, however, surrounded by RER and a typical nucleolar channel system are more frequently observed when progesterone levels are high and the E_2/P ratio low. Junctional complexes appear to be different with respect to progesterone secretion. During the follicular phase and in anovulatory cycles, desmosomes are more abundant and are mainly localized in the apical region of the lateral cell membrane. They are also present in small numbers along the remaining lateral surface. In the luteal phase, these desmosomes seem to disappear in the mid and basal parts of the lateral cell membrane. At the same time, the intercellular space between adjacent epithelial cells becomes larger, mainly at the basal pole. Loose interdigitations of the membrane are observed in the mid and basal part of the lateral wall (FIG. 2). Such epithelial dissociation might favor trophoblastic invasion. High E_2/P ratio and/or low progesterone levels are associated with the presence of numerous desmosomes, less marked membrane interdigitations, and an intercellular space that is not enlarged. In artificial cycles obtained in premature ovarian failure, giant mitochrondria and the nucleolar channel system were only observed when high estradiol doses were administered in the first part of the cycle. This finding points again to the importance of adequate estradiol secretion in the proliferative phase, probably in relation to the synthesis of sufficient progesterone receptors.

In conclusion, our data confirm the normal ultrastructural maturation of the endometrial epithelium after ovarian stimulation. Advanced endometrial maturation occurs in relation to higher progesterone levels. When the E_2/P ratio is elevated, however, abnormal endometrial evolution may be observed. It is difficult to visualize how accelerated endometrial maturation might be favorable to implantation in IVF trials where embryos are replaced in the uterus at 48 hours before the physiological timing.

Attention has been focused on the possible role of surface carbohydrates of both uterine epithelium and trophoblast in implantation. It has been suggested that hormonally induced modifications of these carbohydrates might be important in implantation in rats and mice.[35,36] No changes, however, have been noted so far in the absolute amount of neutral carbohydrates,[35,37] although intraluminal instillation of concanavalin A (Con A) prevents implantation[38] while at the same time inducing decidualization.[39]

In the human, we could not show any changes in endometrial Con A

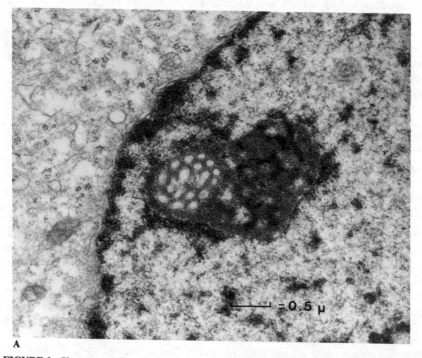

A

FIGURE 2. Characteristic features observed in clomiphene/human menopausal gonadotropin/human chorionic gonadotropin-treated cycles in which high P level and low E_2/P ratios were obtained. **A:** nucleolar channel system; **B:** giant mitochondria; **C:** loose lateral interdigitations.

binding between follicular, early, and late luteal phases. In artificial cycles, however, obtained by giving a sequence of estradiol followed by estradiol with progesterone, in patients suffering from premature ovarian failure,[40] we did not observe any Con A binding. This lack might be due to insufficient estrogenic stimulation, because some of these patients had been amenorrheic for months or years and received only weak doses of estradiol for the first 14 days of the cycle.

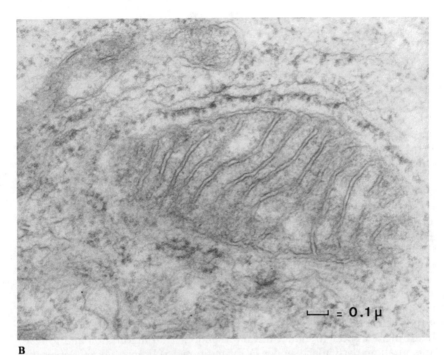

B

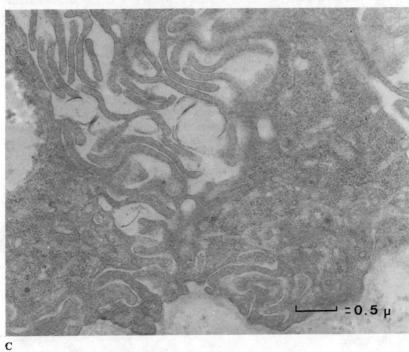

C

FIGURE 2B and C. See legend on p. 70.

CONCLUSIONS

In most species, the uterus plays a major role in the recognition of pregnancy. Secretion of prostaglandins by the uterus in the absence of implantation induces luteolysis, whereas in the presence of implantation sites, this secretion is prevented and luteolysis does not occur. In the human, the role of the uterus in the rescue of the corpus luteum remains doubtful and appears to have been taken over by secretion of hCG by the blastocyst, even perhaps before implantation. The rate of hCG rise seems to have a prognostic value for the rescue of the human corpus luteum.

Finally, extrapolation of animal investigations and comparison with available human data suggest the following: 1) A relative synchronism between embryo and endometrium must be achieved for successful implantation in all species, but less stringent conditions may be required in the human. 2) The uterine receptivity window is well-defined in some laboratory species. In the human this window extends over six days, but evolutive pregnancies seem to be obtained only if implantation takes place on days 5 to 7. 3) Estrogen of the luteal phase triggers implantation in rats and mice by mainly acting at the epithelial level; other species do not necessarily need estrogen at this moment. In the human, however, implantation might be related to critical values of the E_2/P ratio. 4) High progesterone levels in the early human luteal phase appear to induce advanced endometrial maturation and to favor implantation, particularly under IVF conditions. 5) In humans and laboratory rodents, adequate E_2 priming during the follicular phase appears necessary to obtain complete differentiation during the luteal phase.

REFERENCES

1. NOYES, R. W., Z. DICKMAN, L. L. DAYLE & A. M. GATES. 1963. Ovum transfers, synchronous and asynchronous, in the study of implantation. In Delayed Implantation. A. C. Enders, Ed.: 27-35. Univ. Chicago.

2. OGURI, N., Y. TSUTSUMI. 1982. Non-surgical transfer of equine embryos. In In vitro fertilization and embryo transfer. E. S. E. Hafez & K. Sem, Eds.: 287-295. MTP Press Ltd. Lancaster, U.K.

3. LAWSON, R. A. S. 1977. In Embryo transfer in Farm Animals. K. H. Betteridge. Monograph 16. Agriculture Canada. 72-78.

4. LENTON, E. & C. COLMAN. 1985. Critical factors for successful human implantation. First meeting of the European Society of Human Reproduction and Embryology. Bonn, June 23-26.

5. ENGLERT, Y., M. ROYER, J. BELAISCH, M. JONDET, R. FRYDMAN & J. TESTART. 1984. Delayed appearance of plasmatic chorionic gonatropin in pregnancies after in vitro fertilization and embryo transfer. Fertil. Steril. 42: 835-838.

6. FINN, C. A. 1977. The implantation reaction. In Biology of the Uterus. R. M. Wynn, Ed.: 245-308. Plenum Press. New York.

7. MCLAREN, A. 1973. Blastocyst activation. In Regulation of mammalian reproduction. S. J. Segal, R. Crozier, P. A. Corfman & P. G. Condliffe, Eds.: 321-328. Ch. E. Thomas. Springfield.

8. HEALD, P. J. 1976. Biochemical aspects of implantation. J. Reprod. Fertil. Suppl. 25: 29-52.
9. SEGAL, J., W. SCHER & S. S. KOIDE. 1977. Estrogens, nucleic acids and protein synthesis in uterine metabolism. *In* Biology of the uterus. R. W. Wynn, Ed.: 139-201. Plenum Press. New York.
10. LEJEUNE, B., F. PUISSANT, M. CAMUS & F. LEROY. 1982. Induction of implantation in the rat by intraparametrial injection of uterine RNA from oestrogen-treated animals. J. Endocrinol. 93: 397-402.
11. SURANI, M. A. H. 1977. Radiolabelled rat uterine luminal proteins and their regulation by oestradiol and progesterone. J. Reprod. Fertil. 50: 289-296.
12. KIRBY, D. R. S. 1965. The invasiveness of the trophoblast. *In* The early conceptus, normal and abnormal. W. W. Park, Ed.: 68-73. E. S. Livingstone. Edinburgh.
13. FINN, C. A. 1974. The induction of implantation in mice by actinomycin D. J. Endocrinol. 60: 199-200.
14. AITKEN, R. J. 1977. The influence of actinomycin D on the composition of mouse uterine flushings. J. Reprod. Fertil. 50: 193-195.
15. CAMUS, M., B. LEJEUNE & F. LEROY. 1979. Induction of implantation in the rat by intraparametrial injection of actinomycin D. Biol. Reprod. 20: 1115-1118.
16. WEITLAUF, H. M. 1976. Effects of uterine flushings on RNA synthesis by implanting and delayed-implanting mouse blastocysts. Biol. Reprod., 14: 566-571.
17. O'NEILL, C. & P. QUINN. 1981. Interaction of uterine flushings with mouse blastocysts *in vitro* as assessed by the incorporation of ^{3}H uridine. J. Reprod. Fertil. 62: 257-262.
18. LEJEUNE, B., F. LAMY, R. LECOCQ, J. DESCHACHT & F. LEROY. 1985. Patterns of protein synthesis in endometrial tissues from ovariectomized rats treated with estradiol and progesterone. J. Reprod. Fertil. 73: 223-228.
19. FINN, C. A. & L. MARTIN. 1974. The control of implantation. J. Reprod. Fertil. 39: 195-206.
20. LEROY, F., G. SCHETGEN & M. CAMUS. 1980. Initiation of implantation at the subcellular level. Prog. Reprod. Biol. 7: 200-215.
21. PSYCHOYOS, A. 1973. Hormonal control of ovo-implantation. Vitam. Horm. 31: 201-256.
22. LEROY, F., J. VAN HOECK & B. LEJEUNE. 1979. Effect of cycloheximide on the uterine refractory state induced by nidation estrogen in rats. J. Reprod. Fertil. 56: 187-191.
23. YOCHIM, J. M. & R. C. MALLONEE. 1980. Hormonal control of pyridine nucleotideactivity in the uterus: a model for progestational differentiation. Biol. Reprod. 23: 595-605.
24. LEROY, F. & M. CAMUS. 1981. The hormonal regulation of implantation. Acta Europ. Fertil. 12: 187-192.
25. LENTON, E. A., R. SULAIMAN, O. SOBOWALE & I. D. COOKS. 1982. The human menstrual cycle: plasma concentration of prolactin, LH, FSH, oestradiol and progesterone in conceiving and nonconceiving women. J. Reprod. Fertil. 65: 131-139.
26. KARSH, F. J., L. C. KREY, R. F. WEICK, D. J. DIERSAHKE & E. KNOBIL. 1973. Functional luteolysis in the rhesus monkey: the role of estrogen. Endocrinology, 92: 1148-1152.
27. BOARD, J. A., A. S. BHATNAGAR & C. W. BUSH. 1973. Effect of oral diethylstilbestrol on plasma progesterone. Fertil. Steril. 24: 95-99.
28. LEHMAN, F., I. JUST-NASTANSKY, B. BEHRENDT, P. J. CRYGAN & B. BETTENDORF. 1975. Effect of post ovulatory administered oestrogens on corpus luteum function. Acta Endocrinol. (Copenhagen) 79: 329.
29. QUIGLEY, M. M. 1984. The use of ovulation-inducing agents in *in vitro* fertilization. Clin. Obstet. Gynecol. 27 (4).
30. GORDON, M. 1975. Cyclic changes in the fine structure of the epithelial cells of human endometrium. Int. Rev. Cytol. 42: 127-172.
31. MURPHY, C. R., J. G. SWIFT, J. A. NEED, T. M. MUKHERJEE & A. W. ROGERS. 1982. A freeze-fracture electron microscopic study of tight junction epithelial cells in the human uterus. Anat. Embryol. 163: 367-370.
32. SUNDSTROM, P., O. NILSON & P. LIEDHOLM. 1983. Scanning electron microscopy of human preimplantation endometrium in normal and clomid-hMG stimulated cycle. Fertil. Steril. 40: 642-647.
33. GARCIA, J. E., A. A. ACOSTA, J. G. HSIU & H. W. JONES. 1984. Advanced endometrial maturation after ovulation induction with human menopausal gonadotropin/human choronic gonadotropin for *in vitro* fertilization. Fertil. Steril. 41: 31-35.

34. COHEN, J., C. DEBACHE, F. PIGEAU, G. MANDELBAUM, M. PLACHOT & J. DE BRUX. 1984. Sequential use of clomiphene citrate, human menopausal gonadotropin and human chorionic gonadotropin in human *in vitro* fertilization. II Study of luteal phase adequacy following aspiration of the preovulatory follicules. Fertil. Steril. **42:** 360-365.
35. ENDERS, A. C. & S. SCHLAFKE. 1974. Surface coats of the mouse blastocyst and uterus during the preimplantation period. Anat. Rec. **180:** 31-46.
36. SCHLAFKE, S. & A. C. ENDERS. 1975. Cellular basis of interaction between trophoblast and uterus at implantation. Biol. Reprod. **12:** 41-65.
37. MURPHY, C. R. & A. W. ROGERS. 1981. Effects of ovarian hormones on cell membranes in the rat uterus: The surface carbohydrates at the apex of the luminal epithelium. Cell. Biophysics **13:** 305-320.
38. HICKS, J. J. & A. M. GUZMAN-GONZALEZ. 1979. Inhibition of implantation by intraluminal instillation of concanavalin A in mice. Contraception **20:** 129-136.
39. BUXTON, L. E. & N. R. MURDOCH. 1982. Lectins, calcium ionophore A 23187 and peanut oil as deciduogenic agents in the uterus of pseudopregnant mice: effects of tranylcypromine, indomethacin, iproniazid and propanol. Aust. J. Biol. Sci. **35:** 63-72.
40. LUTJEN, P., A. TROUNSON, J. LENTON, J. FINDLAY, C. WOOD & P. RENOU. 1984. The establishment and maintenance of pregnancy using *in vitro* fertilization and embryo donation in a patient with primary ovarian failure. Nature **307:** 174-175.

Primary Culture of Mouse Endometrium on Floating Collagen Gels: A Potential *in Vitro* Model for Implantation[a]

J. SENGUPTA,[b] R. L. GIVEN,[c] J. B. CAREY,[d] AND
H. M. WEITLAUF[d,e]

[b]Department of Physiology
All India Institute of Medical Sciences
New Delhi, 110029, India

[c]Department of Anatomy
University of Texas Medical Branch
Galveston, Texas 77550

[d]Department of Cell Biology and Anatomy
Texas Tech University Health Sciences Center
Lubbock, Texas 79430

INTRODUCTION

In attempting to overcome problems associated with studying implantation in intact animals, several tissue culture systems have been devised in which blastocysts are able to attach to an artificial substratum *in vitro*. Over the past 20 years a variety of substrates have been used in these so-called "*in vitro* models for implantation" including strips of rabbit endometrium[1,2] and whole uteri from immature mice[3,4] maintained as organ cultures; plastic and glass cover slips;[5-11] various types of extracellular matrix material;[12-14] monolayers of "feeder cells" from endometrial and nonendometrial sources;[11,15] and even vesicles of uterine epithelium incubated in hanging drops.[16,17] Enders *et al.*[18] have reviewed what has been learned about the process of trophoblast attachment in most of these *in vitro* systems and critically compared it with what is known about the process as it occurs *in utero*. They concluded that although each of these approaches may be useful for examining some aspect of the interaction between the embryo and its surroundings in the peri-

[a]This work was supported by Grant HD17437-02 from the National Institute of Child Health and Human Development.

[e]To whom correspondence should be addressed.

implantation period, all are limited in one way or another as models of implantation. For example, it was of concern that blastocysts attached to acellular clots and areas of degenerating stroma as well as to the epithelium in the organ cultures and that there was a lack of endocrine specificity. Thus, in these organ cultures, at least, the processes of attachment and penetration were seen as not being precisely the same as those that occur *in vivo*. Similarly, although attachment and outgrowth of trophoblast on plastic or extracellular matrix materials appears to correlate with some developmental changes that occur in embryos at the time of implantation *in vivo*,[19-23] it is obvious that there is not a progressive interaction between embryo and substrate in these situations. Furthermore, the use of cellular monolayers as living substrates has not solved this problem because rather than interacting progressively with the cells, the embryos typically displace them and attach preferentially to the underlying plastic or glass, again without hormone specificity.[6,11,15]

Based on this analysis, it was suggested by Enders and his colleagues that there can never be a totally appropriate *in vitro* model for implantation.[6] Although this is technically correct, the fact remains that it is difficult or impossible to manipulate conditions at the site of embryo attachment *in utero* and therefore, in order to carry out many of the needed studies on implantation, *in vitro* systems should be devised that mimic as closely as possible the interaction of blastocyst and endometrium.

It has recently been realized that many cell types have enhanced proliferation and/or improved morphological as well as biochemical differentiation when grown on collagen as opposed to plastic or glass.[24-27] In some cases these methods have made it possible to maintain primary cultures for prolonged periods in serum-free medium and thus to study the direct effects of various hormones on the cells.[28-30] Although details of the procedures vary with the laboratory and the tissue being studied, two general points emerge from this work. The first is that differentiation of epithelium *in vitro* depends on cells being able to assume a more or less normal shape. For example, mammary epithelium grown as a squamous monolayer on plastic or a rigid collagen matrix shows increased proliferation and decreased synthesis of protein as compared to fresh tissue, and it will not respond to lactogenic hormones. When grown on flexible collagen gels, however, the epithelial cells become cuboidal to columnar in shape and develop "polarity". They stop proliferating and increase protein synthesis, and they are able to respond to lactogenic hormones with secretion of casein. Indeed, it appears that the amount of casein produced is directly related to cell height.[24,31,32] That it is flexibility of the substratum that is essential is shown by the observation that cells grown on collagen that is fixed to the surface of the dish appear to be similar in most ways to those on glass, but when the gels are freed and allowed to contract, the cells reassume a normal shape and again have the ability to respond to lactogenic hormones.[32] Similar observations have been reported with epithelial cells from salivary gland[34] and liver.[28,29]

The second point to be made from the work with collagen is that although normal morphology seems to be necessary for typical epithelial responses to hormones, it is not always sufficient. For example, uterine and vaginal epithelium grown on collagen have a normal appearance and even contain characteristic populations of hormone receptors, but they do not respond to estrogen *in vitro*.[35,36] Thus, there is a growing awareness that stroma and epithelium may have to interact for some tissues to react to steroid hormones, and that this requirement may be particularly important in the reproductive tract.[37] Indeed, it has been reported that when gels containing vaginal or uterine epithelium are transplanted to the kidney of intact females they will respond to endogenous estrogen only if they contain appropriate stromal elements as well.[38] From this it might be anticipated that in order to develop a hormone-responsive *in vitro* model for implantation it will be critical to have not only a normal-appearing epithelium but also to have it in contact with uterine stroma.

The purpose of the present communication is to present the results of our preliminary attempts to develop an *in vitro* model of implantation consisting of such an "endometrium". We have used dissociated cells from the uteri of adult mice as the starting material and have cultured them on a flexible three-dimensional substratum of reconstituted mouse tail collagen.

MATERIAL AND METHODS

A modification of the procedure developed for culturing mammary gland tissue[24] was used in our pilot studies to determine the feasibility of using reconstituted collagen as a substratum for endometrial cells. The steps taken in preparation of collagen gels and dissociation of endometrial cells are briefly as follows.

Preparation of Collagen Gels

Approximately 6 gr of mouse tail collagen fibers were dissolved overnight in 300 ml 0.5 M acetic acid; the supernatant after centrifugation at 12,500 $\times$ g for 1 h was decanted into dialysis tubing (12,000-14,000 mw cutoff) and dialyzed against 2 liters of 10% medium 199 (M 199, Grand Island Biological Company [Gibco], Grand Island, New York, USA) for 24 h at 4° C (this was repeated once) to provide the stock collagen solution. The stock solution was diluted to the desired concentration with sterile distilled water, and one volume was added to 0.3 volumes of a solution containing 0.14 M NaOH and 10 $\times$ M 199 (1:1 vol/vol) and kept on ice to prevent gelation.

Dissociation of Endometrium and Preparation Cells

Approximately 1 gr whole uteri (from sexually mature Swiss-Webster mice at random stages of the estrous cycle) was placed in 10 ml Hank's

Balanced Salt Solution (HBSS pH 7.2-7.4, Gibco) with a mixture of proteolytic enzymes and albumin (50 mg pronase, Calbiochem-Behring [Calbiochem], La Jolla, California, USA; 25 mg collagenase, Boehringer-Mannheim Biochemicals [Boehringer], Indianapolis, Indiana, USA, grade 2; and 25 mg bovine serum albumin, crystalized, BSA, Sigma [Sigma], St. Louis, Missouri, USA), minced with fine scissors, and incubated for 1 h at 37° C in a shaking water bath. The resulting cell suspension was filtered through sterile gauze and centrifuged at 500 $\times$ g for 10 min; the pellet was resuspended in 6 ml HBSS and centrifuged again at 500 $\times$ g for 5 minutes. The cells were resuspended in 5 ml HBSS containing DNase (20 μg/ml, type I, Sigma) and incubated for 30 min at 37° C. The resulting cell suspension was centrifuged at 600 $\times$ g for 5 min, and the pellet was resuspended in 1.0 ml HBSS; this was placed on a 40% colloidal silica coated with polyvinyl pyrrolidone (Percoll; Pharmacia Fine Chemicals, Piscataway, New Jersey, USA) gradient and centrifuged at 600 $\times$ g for 20 min at room temperature. Cells at the interface were resuspended in 5 ml HBSS and centrifuged 600 $\times$ g for 5 min; this step was repeated, and the pellet was resuspended in 1 ml medium to determine cell number and viability by trypan blue exclusion.

Two different procedures were employed from this point onward. 1) In the initial studies, cells were plated onto the surface of polymerized collagen gels. In this case approximately 300 μl of the collagen solution was spread evenly in 16 mm chambers of multiwell tissue culture plates (Falcon, Division of Becton Dickinson Company, Oxnard, California, USA) and allowed to polymerize at room temperature (0.5 h). The gels were washed with M 199 containing insulin 5 μg/ml, transferrin 5 ng/ml, and selenium 5 ng/ml, (ITS, Collaborative Research Incorporated [Collaborative Research], Lexington, Massachusetts, USA) and stored until use at 37° C in M 199 with ITS and antibiotics (penicillin, 100 units/ml; streptomycin, 100 μg/ml; and Fungizone, 0.25 μg/ml; Gibco). The cell concentration was adjusted to 1 $\times$ 10^6 cells/ml with M 199 containing ITS, antibiotics, and 10% fetal bovine serum (Gibco), and 1 ml of the cell suspension was layered onto the polymerized collagen. 2) For other experiments, the cells were embedded within the collagen gel. This was done by mixing the cell suspension with solubilized collagen to give final concentrations of 1.02 mg of collagen and 1.5 $\times$ 10^6 cells/ml; 300 μl of this mixture was plated in each chamber of a 24 multiwell plate and allowed to polymerize at room temperature. Approximately 1 ml of serum-free M 199 supplemented with ITS, antibiotics, fibroblast growth factor (FGF, 10 ng/ml, Collaborative Research), cholera toxin (10 ng/ml, Calbiochem), and BSA were added, and the gels were incubated at 37° C in 5% CO_2 in air. The gels were freed with a sterile spatula and gentle shaking at 24 h and moved to 35 mm culture dishes in 1 ml of supplemented serum-free medium. At intervals of 2 days, gels were selected and dissolved with collagenase (1% in HBSS), and cell counts were done in the standard way with a hemocytometer. In some cases, a second seeding of cells was placed on the gels, and epidermal growth factor (EGF, 10 ng/ml, Collaborative Research) was added. In a few cultures estradiol 17β (1 $\times$ 10^{-9} M) or progesterone (1 $\times$ 10^{-6} M) were added to the medium.

Fixation and Embedding

Gels were fixed for microscopy with 2.5% glutaraldehyde in 0.1 M sodium cacodylate buffer (pH 7.2) for 2 h at room temperature, rinsed with 0.1 M cacodylate buffer, and postfixed for 1 h with 1% osmium (in the same buffer). Some gels were dehydrated, critical point dried, and gold coated for viewing in the scanning electron microscope (Hitachi 500, Hitachi Scientific Instruments Divison, Mountain View, California, USA). The remainder of the gels were dehydrated, embedded in epon-araldite mixture, and sections were cut perpendicular to the surface layer. Thick sections (1 μm) were stained with 1% toluidene blue and examined by light microscopy; thin sections (silver) were stained with uranyl acetate and lead citrate and examined in the transmission electron microscope (Phillips 300, Phillips Instruments, Holland).

RESULTS

Endometrium Plated onto Collagen Gels

Viability of the cells after dissociation of endometrium with this procedure was typically between 85 and 90%, and most of the cells appeared to be attached to the gel surface within 18-20 h after seeding. Two types of cells could be distinguished by phase microscopy: rounded cells that tended to aggregate and were presumed to be epithelial, and flattened stellate cells, presumed to be fibroblasts. Upon becoming detached from the multi-well plates, the gels would float and immediately begin to contract and fold upon themselves. By the fourth day it was seen that there were patches of epithelial cells on the surface. (Figures 1-7 show examples of cell types present when cells were placed on the surface of polymerized collagen.) In some areas the cells appeared to be attached directly to the collagen (FIG. 1); in others they appeared to be associated with fibroblasts just beneath the surface of the gel (FIG. 2). With the scanning electron microscope it could be seen that these cells were rounded and had numerous microvilli (FIG. 3); in some areas small blebs or larger bulbous projections were observed (FIG. 4). By day 6 of culture, the surface cells tended to be cuboidal or low columnar in shape. They had either central or basal nuclei, and with the transmission electron microscope, evidence of polarization was observed. The apical borders facing the medium were covered with microvilli having a prominent glycocalyx, and the lateral borders were characterized by some interdigitating processes and apical junctional complexes. These cells also contained numerous lipid droplets and large apical vesicles characteristic of uterine epithelium *in vivo;* abundant polysomes, typical mitochondria, and rough endoplasmic reticulum (RER) were also present (FIG. 5). Although a basal lamina was not apparent, there was a close association of the basal border of the cells with collagen fibrils of the matrix

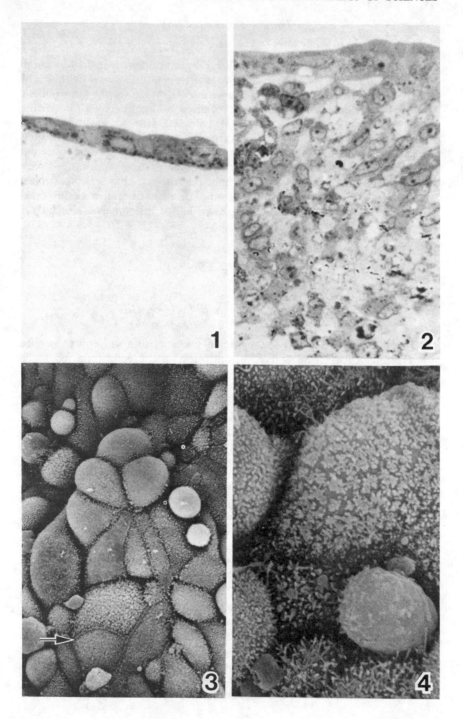

(FIG. 6). The second cell type, typically found beneath the surface layer, had fine processes extending into the surrounding matrix and bore a structural similarity to fibroblasts found in uterine stroma (FIG. 7).

The results of these pilot studies demonstrated that dissociated uterine cells obtained from adult mice will organize on a collagen gel into an endometrium-like complex with a polarized epithelium associated, in some areas at least, with subjacent stromal cells. Although this was encouraging, and made it seem likely that such tissue-like complexes could be used for studying some aspects of implantation *in vitro,* the uneven contraction and extensive folding of the gels presented a problem. Indeed, with cultures of more than a week, the surface epithelium was most often completely inside the gel, and although there were areas of epithelium that appeared histologically normal, the cells were not readily accessible for manipulation. Therefore, in the remaining experiments, cells were embedded within the collagen before polymerization so the contraction would be more uniform[38] and provide a convex surface for the epithelium.

Endometrial Cells Embedded Within Collagen Gels

Collagen containing a mixture of endometrial cells was typically found to be polymerized within 30 min at room temperature, and the cells were effectively embedded within the matrix. As the gels were freed and moved to 35 mm culture plates (at 24 h), they began to contract. The average number of cells per gel was found to decrease from 4.5×10^5 to approximately 1×10^4 during the first five or six days and remained nearly constant for the next week or 10 days. As in the previous experiments, stellate cells resembling fibroblasts and rounded epithelial cells were observed. (Figures 8-13 show examples of cell types present in gels when cells were embedded within the collagen.) The stellate cells were scattered throughout the gel and appeared healthy, whereas those rounded cells within the gels appeared to be degenerating. Considerable debris was present (FIG. 8). Stellate cells dominated the interior of the gels and were found to be more fusiform in shape near

---

FIGURE 1. Light micrograph of cuboidal epithelial cells on a collagen gel. Numerous lipid droplets are present throughout the cytoplasm. Note the absence of cells within the gel and compare this to FIGURE 2; ($\times$ 800).

FIGURE 2. Light micrograph of cuboidal to low columnar cells on the surface of a collagen gel. These cells have round to oval nuclei with prominent nucleoli and lipid droplets. Beneath the epithelium, numerous cells have invaded the gel to form a stroma. These cells are stellate or fusiform in shape and have an oval nucleus with prominent nucleolus; ($\times$ 800).

FIGURE 3. Scanning electron micrograph of the apical surface of epithelial cells on a collagen gel, showing rounded surfaces with numerous short microvilli. In the lower portion of the micrograph the line of attachment of adjacent epithelial cells (arrow) is visible; ($\times$ 1000).

FIGURE 4. Higher magnification micrograph of the surface of the epithelial cells showing the short dense microvilli; spherical protrusions are also associated with the surface of these cells; ($\times$ 4000).

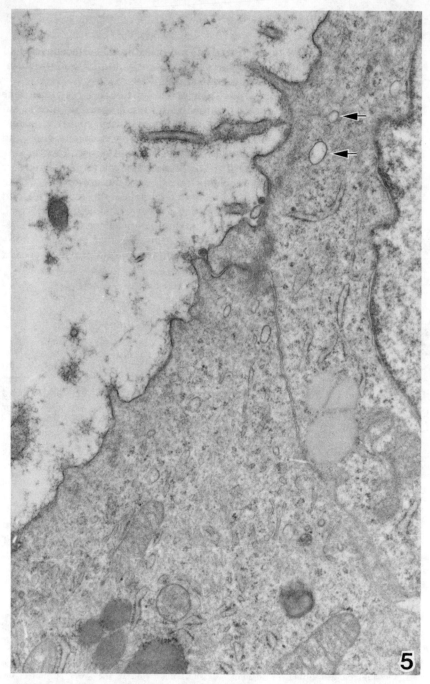

FIGURE 5. A junctional complex is present between these two epithelial cells. The cytoplasm contains short cisternae of rough and smooth endoplasmic reticulum (ER), lipid droplets, small vesicular profiles, and some larger apical vesicles (arrows). Microfilaments occupy the area just beneath the apical cell membrane; short microvilli protrude from the surface with its prominent glycocalyx; ($\times$ 25,800).

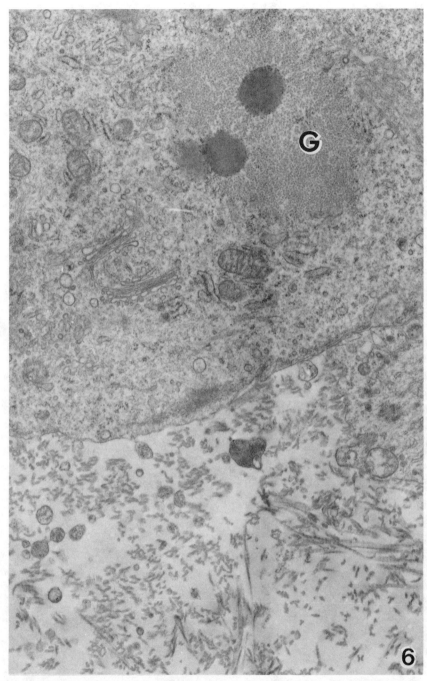

FIGURE 6. Basal surface of an epithelial cell closely associated with collagen of the gel; no basal lamina has developed. A Golgi complex, polysomes, short cisternae of rough and smooth ER, and lipid droplets are visible in the cytoplasm. The accumulation of glycogen (G) seen here was not common in these epithelial cells; ($\times$ 20,400).

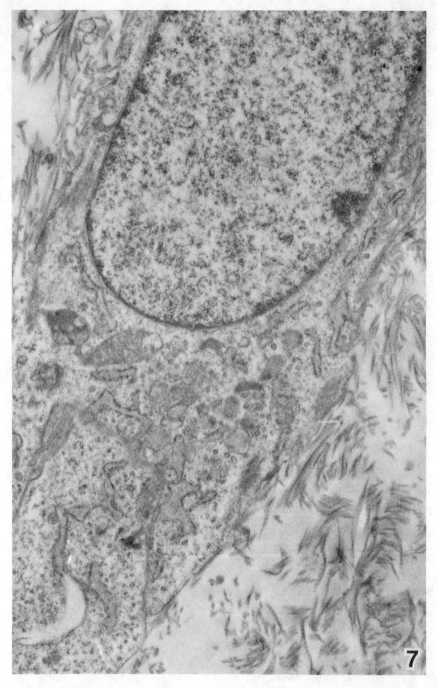

FIGURE 7. Collagen fibers are closely associated with this fibroblast in the stroma of an endometrial construct; a Golgi complex and numerous polysomes are also present in the cytoplasm. The cisternae of the RER are filled with an electron dense material; (× 20,400).

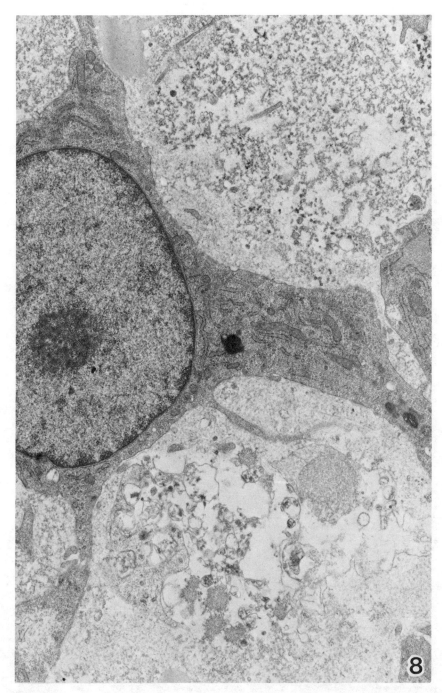

FIGURE 8. This stellate fibroblast embedded in the stroma is surrounded by debris formed by degeneration of cells during contraction of the gel. Numerous cisternae of RER filled with electron dense material can be seen, and there is a prominent nucleolus; ($\times$ 9,800).

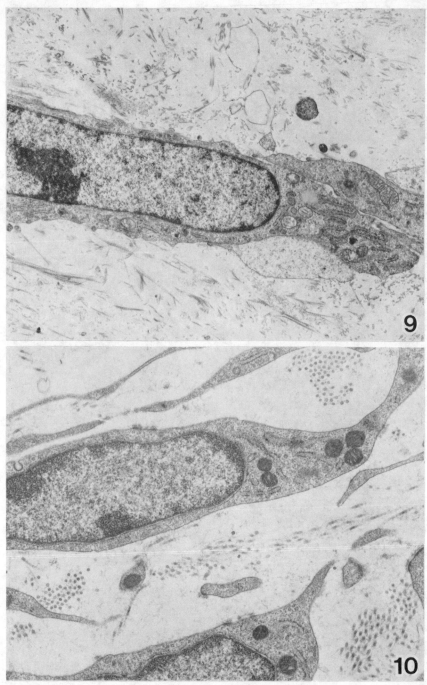

FIGURE 9. A fusiform stromal cell is closely associated with collagen fibers. An elongate nucleus with a prominent nucleolus, numerous cisternae of RER, and a lipid droplet (arrow) are present; ($\times$ 9,000).

FIGURE 10. Fibroblast found in the endometrial stroma of a castrate animal. It contains cisternae of RER, mitochondria, and a prominent nucleolus and differs little from the fibroblasts *in vitro* shown in FIGURES 7, 8, and 9.

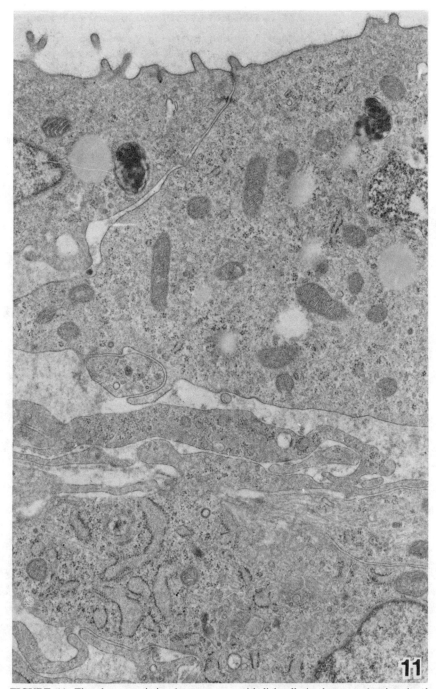

FIGURE 11. The close association between two epithelial cells is shown, and a junctional complex is present at the apical surface. Short microvilli and a prominent glycocalyx are found along the apical cell membrane. Short cisternae of RER, numerous polysomes, lipid droplets, and phagolysosomes are found in the cytoplasm; note the lack of an epithelial basal lamina. Stromal cells are closely associated with the base of the epithelial cells. Slightly dilated cisternae of RER filled with electron dense material are present in the stromal cells; (× 18,400).

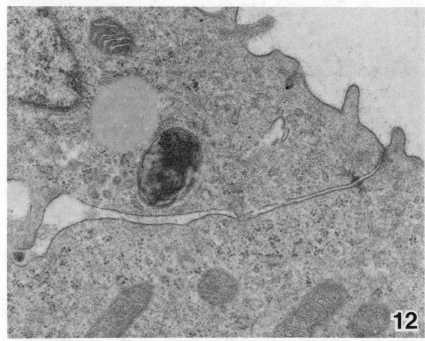

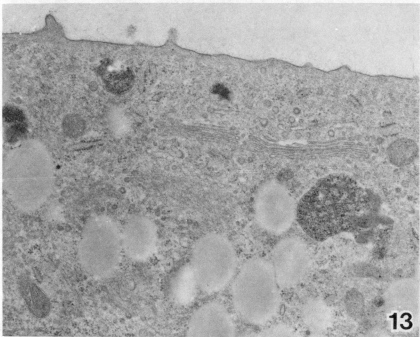

the surface. These cells had a round nucleus with a prominent nucleolus, numerous free polysomes, and interconnecting cisternae of the RER. The cisternae were dilated and filled with electron dense material. Occasionally, lipid droplets or a Golgi complex was seen in the cytoplasm. The processes of these fibroblast-like cells often contacted adjacent cells, although no distinct surface specializations were observed (FIGS. 8-9). These cells were very similar in appearance to those observed in stroma of intact endometrium (compare FIGS. 7, 8, and 9 with 10). By the fifth day the gels became more compacted, fibroblasts appeared to be organizing in layers near the surface, and there were occasional rounded epithelium-like cells on the surface. Except for continued contraction, and the consequent increase in density of cell packing, the gels remained unchanged for as long as 20-30 days in culture.

Rounded cells were typically very scarce on the surface unless a second seeding was done. Then extensive areas were found to be covered with cells, although they did not form a complete layer around the gel. As in the earlier experiments, these surface cells were cuboidal to low columnar in shape with a central round to oval nucleus and a prominent nucleolus. Their apical surfaces were covered with a visible glycocalyx and short microvilli. Adjacent cells had extensive parallel lateral borders with apparent junctional complexes, including desmosomes, at the apical end and extensive interdigitation of the basolateral regions. The cytoplasm typically contained numerous free polysomes, short cisternae of RER, numerous small vesicles, and a Golgi complex near the apical surface; lipid droplets and apical vesicle profiles were also seen (FIGS. 11-13). In addition to the obvious polarization of the cells, the absence of extensive interconnected RER helped to distinguish them from the underlying stromal cells. The basal surfaces of the epithelial cells were rounded with no distinct surface specializations. Stromal cells were found adjacent to epithelium and followed the contour of the basal surface of those cells, but there was no direct contact and no evidence of basal lamina formation (FIG. 11).

Gels incubated for more than seven days in medium containing estradiol appeared to have more extensive areas of surface covered with epithelium than did those incubated with progesterone.

DISCUSSION

The results of these preliminary experiments demonstrate that dissociated mouse "endometrium" will reorganize on floating collagen gels in vitro to

FIGURE 12. Higher magnification of the junctional complex shown in FIGURE 11. It consists of a very close approximation of the apicolateral cell membrane and a desmosome. Numerous polysomes, small apical vesicles, lipid droplets, and a phagolysosome are present. A prominent glycocalyx covers the microvilli and apical cell membrane; ($\times$ 32,900).

FIGURE 13. A prominent Golgi complex and numerous small vesicles are present in the apical portion of this epithelial cell. Numerous lipid droplets, phagolysosomes, and polysomes are also present; ($\times$ 22,400).

form tissue-like masses consisting of a stromal core and a surface layer of epithelium. The stroma and epithelium in these endometrium-like constructs have morphologic similarities to their counterparts *in vivo* and can be maintained in serum-free medium for more than three weeks. The long-term maintenance *in vitro* of uterine epithelium with differentiated characteristics is in marked contrast to the rapid loss of normal morphologic features that occurs when dissociated endometrium is cultured on plastic.[11] Hence, the experience with endometrium is similar to that reported for many tissues including mammary gland,[32] salivary gland,[33] liver,[27] and vagina.[34] Because it is now generally recognized that the ability of many endocrine-sensitive tissues to respond to hormones *in vitro* depends on the maintenance of normal morphological characteristics, and/or interaction between stromal and epithelial cells, we expect that such endometrial constructs will provide an improvement over current *in vitro* models for studies on implantation.

Although development of "endometrium" on collagen gels appears to hold promise for the development of an experimental model, several problems must be solved before it can be used to study the process of implantation. For example, contraction of the gel is uneven when cells are plated only on the upper surface, and this tends to cause them to fold upon themselves and sequester the epithelium. Casting cells into the collagen before it polymerizes effectively overcomes the problem of folding, because the contraction is more uniform, but the gels still shrink to approximately one-eighth of their original size. Bell *et al.*[38] have been successful in regulating the amount of contraction in gels containing epidermal fibroblasts by varying either the amount of collagen or the concentration of cells, and it seems probable that endometrial constructs will behave similarly. Embedding cells within the gels solved the problem of folding, but embedding presented other difficulties. First, epithelial cells that were embedded in the gel typically degenerated within a few days, and occasionally the whole endometrial construct would disintegrate, presumably because of released lysosomal enzymes. This could probably be avoided by separating epithelial and stromal cells before seeding, or by allowing fibroblasts to migrate into the gels from monolayers grown first on plastic as has been done with stroma of both vagina and uterus.[39] The second problem associated with casting cells into the gel was that very few epithelial cells were found on the surface after polymerization and contraction. A two-step procedure, with a secondary seeding of epithelium after contraction of the gel has been used successfully with epidermis,[40] and from the present experience seems to overcome this problem with endometrium as well. Another difficulty with the procedure described here is that although the epithelial cells are cuboidal in shape and appear to be polarized as they are *in vivo*, they are not so regular or as high as they are in the intact uterus. Furthermore, basal lamina is not formed, at least in the first two to three weeks. This may reflect a requirement for additional factors such as fibronectin or laminin, which seem to be necessary for efficient attachment of some epithelial cells to collagen and to enhance formation of basal lamina in constructs of epithelium and stroma similar to those described here.[25,41,42]

In addition to solving these problems, it will be necessary to provide convincing evidence that the epithelium and stroma in these endometrial constructs respond appropriately to ovarian hormones with changes in certain cytological or histochemical features,[43-45] mitotic activity,[46] or the synthesis of various proteins[47] and populations of hormone receptors.[48,49]

Finally, because the most sought-after goal for those interested in *in vitro* models of implantation is to demonstrate hormone-dependent attachment of embryos to uterine epithelium, it seems appropriate to sound a further note of caution. The assumption is that the acid test for *in vitro* models of implantation will be the demonstration that blastocysts (*e.g.,* mouse) do not attach to a progesterone-dominated "endometrium" for some period *in vitro* and that they can then be induced to attach, or implant, at a later time by addition of estrogen. Several points should be made about this expectation. 1) In delayed implanted mice the embryo is metabolically quiescent, and the uterus has reduced sensitivity to a decidualizing stimulus; thus, it seems that down-regulation of both the embryo and the endometrium may be involved in the failure of attachment.[50] 2) We know that delayed implanted embryos become metabolically active when they are placed *in vitro* whether hormones are present or not;[51] we do not know if the endometrial constructs (or other models of "endometrium") will be able to maintain embryos in a metabolically dormant condition *in vitro*. 3) It has been reported that delayed implanted mouse embryos will implant without regard to hormonal conditions in either extra uterine sites,[52,53] or the uterus if the epithelium has been disrupted by a scratch.[54,55] Therefore, if embryos do not remain dormant when incubated *in vitro* with progesterone dominated "endometrium", or if the epithelium on the "endometrium" is incomplete, it might be anticipated that attachment will occur regardless of the hormonal milieu and usefulness of the model, for studies on implantation would be limited. On the other hand, if the embryos do remain quiescent, or if the progesterone-dominated epithelium can resist an active embryo (or both), then it may be possible to achieve a kind of delay of implantation *in vitro*. That would provide an important tool for studying the process of implantation.

In conclusion, it should be emphasized that although these tissue-like complexes may be shown to resemble endometrium in many ways, and although they may be useful for manipulating conditions at the site of embryo attachment and thus for studying some aspects of the interaction between embryo and uterus, they cannot provide an ". . . increasingly intimate interaction of a blastocyst with endometrium of an intact uterus. . .".[18] Therefore, as Enders and his colleagues have already pointed out,[18] such models can never mimic totally the process of implantation.

REFERENCES

1. GLENISTER, T. W. 1963. Observations on mammalian blastocysts implanting in organ culture. *In* Delayed Implantation. A. C. Enders, Ed. University of Chicago Press. Chicago, Il.

2. GLENISTER, T. W. 1966. Nidation processes in organ culture. Int. J. Fertil. **11:** 412-423.
3. GRANT, P. S. 1973. The effect of progesterone and oestradiol on blastocysts cultured within the lumina of immature mouse uteri. J. Embryol. Exp. Morphol. **29:** 617-638.
4. GRANT, P. S., I. LJUNGKVIST & O. NILSSON. 1975. The hormonal control and morphology of blastocyst invasion in the mouse uterus *in vitro.* J. Embryol. Exp. Morphol. **34:** 200-310.
5. MINTZ, B. 1964. Formation of genetically mosaic embryos and early development of "lethal (t^{12}/t^{12})-normal" mosaics. J. Exp. Zool. **157:** 273-292.
6. COLE. R. J. & R. J. PAUL. 1965. Properties of cultured preimplantation mouse and rabbit embryos, and cell strains derived from them. *In* Preimplantation Stages of Pregnancy. G. E. W. Wolstenholme & M. O'Connor, Eds. Academic Press. New York.
7. GWATKIN, R. B. L. 1966. Amino acid requirements for attachment and outgrowth of the mouse blastocyst *in vitro.* J. Cell Physiol. **68:** 335-344.
8. SHERMAN, M. I. 1972. Biochemistry of differentiation of mouse trophoblast: esterase. Exp. Cell Res. **75:** 449-459.
9. SHERMAN, M. I. 1972. Biochemistry of differentiation of mouse trophoblast: alkaline phosphatase. Dev. Biol. **27:** 337-350.
10. SPINDLE, A. I. & R. A. PEDERSEN. 1973. Hatching. attachment, and outgrowth of mouse blastocysts *in vitro:* fixed nitrogen requirements. J. Exp. Zool. **186:** 305-318.
11. SALOMON, D. S. & M. I. SHERMAN. 1975. Implantation and invasiveness of mouse blastocysts on uterine monolayers. Exp. Cell Res. **90:** 261-268.
12. JENKINSON, E. J. & I. B. WILSON. 1970. *In vitro* support systems for the study of blastocyst differentiation in the mouse. Nature (London) **228:** 776-778.
13. JENKINSON, E. J. & I. B. WILSON. 1973. *In vitro* studies on the control of trophoblast outgrowth in the mouse. J. Embryol. Exp. Morphol. **30:** 21-30.
14. GLASS, R. H., J. AGGELER, A. I. SPINDLE, R. A. PEDERSEN & Z. WEBB. 1983. Degradation of extracellular matrix by mouse trophoblast outgrowths: a model for implantation. J. Cell Biol. **96:** 1108-1116.
15. GLASS, R. H., A. I. SPINDLE & R. A. PEDERSEN. 1979. Mouse embryo attachment to substratum and interaction of trophoblast with cultured cells. J. Exp. Zool. **208:** 327-336.
16. MORRIS, J. E., S. W. POTTER & P. M. BUCKLEY. 1982. Mouse embryos and uterine epithelia show adhesive interactions in culture. J. Exp. Zool. **222:** 195-198.
17. MORRIS, J. E., S. W. POTTER, L. RYND & P. M. BUCKLEY. 1983. Adhesion of mouse blastocysts to uterine epithelium in culture: a requirement for mutual surface interactions. J. Exp. Zool. **225:** 467-479.
18. ENDERS, A. C., D. J. CHAVEZ & S. SCHLAFKE. 1981. Comparison of implantation *in utero* and *in vitro. In* Cellular and Molecular Aspects of Implantation. S. R. Glasser & D. W. Bullock, Eds. Plenum Press. New York.
19. ELLUM, K. A. O. & R. B. L. GWATKIN. 1968. Patterns of nucleic acid synthesis in the early mouse embryo. Dev. Biol. **18:** 311-330.
20. SHERMAN, M. I. & D. S. SALOMON. 1975. The relationships between the early mouse embryo and its environment. *In* The Developmental Biology of Reproduction. C. L. Markert & J. Papaconstantinou, Eds. Academic Press. New York.
21. STRICKLAND, S., E. REICH & M. I. SHERMAN. 1976. Plasminogen activator in early embryogenesis: enzyme production by trophoblast and parietal endoderm. Cell **9:** 231-240.
22. JENKINSON, E. J. & R. F. SEARLE. 1977. Cell surface on the mouse blastocyst at implantation. Exp. Cell Res. **106:** 386-390.
23. SHALGI, R. & M. I. SHERMAN. 1979. Scanning electron microscopy of the surface of normal and implantation-delayed mouse blastocysts during development *in vitro.* J. Exp. Zool. **210:** 69-80.
24. EMERMAN, J. T. & D. R. PITELKA. 1977. Maintenance and induction of morphological differentiation in dissociated mammary epithelium on floating collagen membranes. In Vitro **13:** 316-328.
25. GOSPODAROWICZ, D., G. GREENBERG & C. R. BIRDWELL. 1978. Determination of cellular shape by the extracellular matrix and its correlation with the control of cellular growth. Cancer. Res. **38:** 4155-4171.
26. KLEINMAN, H. K., R. J. KLEBE & G. R. MARTIN. 1981. Role of collagenous matrices in the adhesion and growth of cells. J. Cell Biol. **88:** 473-485.

27. HAY, E. D. 1982. Cell-matrix interaction in embryonic avian cornea and lens. *In* Extracellular Matrix. S. P. Hawkes & J. L. Wang, Eds. Academic Press. New York.

28. MICHALOPOULOS, G. & H. C. PITOT. 1975. Primary culture of parenchymal liver cells on collagen membranes. Exp. Cell Res. **94:** 70-78.

29. MICHALOPOULOS, G., G. L. SATTLER & H. C. PITOT. 1978. Hormonal regulation and the effects of glucose on tyrosine aminotransferase activity in adult rat hepatocytes cultured on floating collagen membranes. Cancer Res. **38:** 1550-1555.

30. IMAGAWA, W., Y. TOMOOKA & S. NANDI. 1982. Serum-free growth of normal and tumor mouse mammary epithelial cells in primary culture. Proc. Natl. Acad. Sci. USA **79:** 4074-4077.

31. EMERMAN, J. T., J. ENAMI, D. R. PITELKA & S. NANDI. 1977. Hormonal effects on intracellular and secreted casein in cultures of mouse mammary epithelial cells on floating collagen membranes. Proc. Natl. Acad. Sci. USA **74:** 4466-4470.

32. BURWEN, S. & D. R. PITELKA. 1980. Secretory function of lactating mouse mammary epithelial cells cultured on collagen gels. Exp. Cell Res. **126:** 249-262.

33. SHANNON, J. M. & D. R. PITELKA. 1981. The influence of cell shape on the induction of functional differentiation in mouse mammary cells *in vitro*. In Vitro **17:** 1016-1028.

34. YANG, J., D. FLYNN, L. LARSON & S. HAMAMOTO. 1982. Growth in primary culture of mouse submandibular epithelial cells embedded in collagen gels. In Vitro **18:** 435-442.

35. IGUCHI, T., F-A.D. UCHIMA, P. C. OSTRANDER & H. BERN. 1983. Growth of normal mouse vaginal epithelial cells in and on collagen gels. Proc. Natl. Acad. Sci. USA **80:** 3743-3747.

36. EDERY, M., L. I. SEWELL & H. BERN. 1985. Estrogen induces progestin receptor but not proliferation of mouse endometrial epithelial cells *in vitro*. Endocrinology **116:** Abst. 329.

37. CUNHA, G. R. 1976. Epithelial-stromal interactions in development of the urogenital tract. Int. Rev. Cytol. **47:** 137-194.

38. COOKE, P. S., D. K. FUJII, F-D. A. UCHIMA, L. I. SEWELL, H. BERN & G. R. CUNHA. 1985. Restoration of normal morphology and function in cultured vaginal and uterine epithelia transplanted with stroma *in vivo*. Endocrinology **116:** Abst. 260.

39. BELL, E., B. IVARSSON & C. MERRILL. 1979. Production of a tissue-like structure by contraction of collagen lattices by human fibroblasts of different proliferative potential *in vitro*. Proc. Natl. Acad. Sci. USA **76:** 1274-1278.

40. BELL, E., C. MERRILL & D. SOLOMON. 1979. Characteristics of a tissue-equivalent formed by fibroblasts cast in a collagen gel. J. Cell Biol. **83:** 398 abst.

41. BROWNELL, A. G., C. C. BESSEM & H. C. SLAVKIN. 1981. Possible functions of mesenchyme cell-derived fibronectin during formation of basal lamina. Proc. Natl. Acad. Sci. USA **78:** 3711-3715.

42. GARBI, C. & S. H. WOLLMAN. 1982. Basal lamina formation on thyroid epithelia in separated follicles in suspension culture. J. Cell Biol. **94:** 489-492.

43. ALDEN, R. H. 1947. Implantation of the rat egg. II. Alteration in osmophilic epithelial lipids of the rat uterus under normal and experimental conditions. Anat. Rec. **97:** 1-13.

44. BROKELMANN, J. & D. W. FAWCETT. 1969. The localization of endogenous peroxidase in the rat uterus and its induction by estradiol. Biol. Reprod. **1:** 59-71.

45. NILSSON, O. 1972. Ultrastructure of the process of secretion in the rat uterine epithelium at preimplantation. J. Ultrastruc. Res. **40:** 572-580.

46. FINN, C. A. 1977. The implantation reaction. *In* Biology of the Uterus. R. M. Wynn, Ed. Plenum Press. New York.

47. LEJEUNE, B., F. LAMY, R. LECOCQ, J. DESCHACHT & F. LEROY. 1985. Patterns of protein synthesis in endometrial tissues from ovariectomized rats treated with oestradiol and progesterone. J. Reprod. Fertil. **173:** 223-228.

48. MARKAVERICH, B. M., S. UPCHURCH, S. A. MCCORMACK, S. R. GLASSER & J. H. CLARK. 1981. Differential stimulation of uterine cells by nafoxidine and chlomiphene: relationship between nuclear estrogen receptors and type II estrogen binding sites and cellular growth. Biol. Reprod. **24:** 171-181.

49. SUMIDA, C. & J. R. PASQUALINI. 1980. Dynamic studies on estrogen response in fetal guinea pig uterus: effect of estradiol administration on estradiol receptor, progesterone receptor and uterine growth. J. Recept. Res. **1:** 439-457.

50. McLAREN, A. 1973. Blastocyst activation. *In* The Regulation of Mammalian Reproduction. S. J. Segal, R. Crozier, P. A. Corfman & P. G. Condliffe, Eds. Chas. Thomas Publishers. Springfield, Il.

51. WEITLAUF, H. M. 1973. *In vitro* uptake and incorporation of amino acids by blastocysts from intact and ovariectomized mice. J. Exp. Zool. **183:** 303-308.

52. WEITLAUF, H. M. 1969. Temporal changes in protein synthesis by mouse blastocysts transferred to ovariectomized recipients. J. Exp. Zool. **171:** 481-486.

53. FAWCETT, D., G. B. WISLOCKI & C. M. WALDO. 1947. The development of mouse ova in the anterior chamber of the eye and in the abdominal cavity. Am. J. Anat. **81:** 413-443.

54. KIRBY, D. R. S. 1967. Ectopic autografts of blastocysts in mice maintained in delayed implantation. J. Reprod. Fertil. **14:** 515-517.

55. COWELL, T. P. 1969. Implantation and development of mouse eggs transferred to the uteri of non-progestational mice. J. Reprod. Fertil. **19:** 239-245.

Biochemical Responses of the Luminal Epithelium and Uterine Sensitization[a]

B. C. MOULTON AND B. B. KOENIG

Departments of Obstetrics-Gynecology, Physiology and
Biophysics, and Biochemistry and Molecular Biology
University of Cincinnati College of Medicine
Cincinnati, Ohio 45267-0526

After many years of research in blastocyst implantation, two fundamental questions remain: What is the signal given by the blastocyst to initiate the implantation reaction? and What are the mechanisms by which the uterus receives this signal and responds with the growth and differentiation of the placenta? Our eventual understanding of the initial events of pregnancy and their control will require answers to both of these questions.[1]

During early pregnancy the uterus becomes sensitive to the presence of the blastocyst for only a limited period of time.[2,3] This transitory change in uterine sensitivity presumably depends upon changes in uterine capacity to receive and to respond to the blastocyst signal. The cellular and biochemical bases for uterine sensitivity, however, have been difficult to establish because of the complexities of the system. In addition to the necessary developmental maturity of the embryo, the cellular functions of the luminal and glandular epithelia and the stroma of the endometrium must be coordinated and controlled. Both progesterone and estrogen secretion participate in this coordination and control, and the development and timing of uterine sensitivity depends upon both serum levels and the ratio of progesterone to estrogen. Specific biochemical effects of these hormones on uterine cell types have been identified, but these observations have not yielded a complete explanation for uterine sensitivity.[4-10]

Potential interactions between various uterine cell types during the physiological events of early pregnancy result in further complexities for studies of blastocyst implantation. In several hormonal target organs, the hormonal responses of epithelial cells depend upon an interaction of the epithelium with underlying stromal cells.[11] Evidence suggests that many hormone responses within epithelial cells may not be elicited directly in these cells, but instead may be elicited by putative growth factors or inductors elaborated in neigh-

[a]NIH Grants HD-07255 and HD-10721 provided support for the author's research.

95

boring stromal cells in response to hormonal stimulation. The hormonal control of morphogenesis, therefore, becomes dependent upon more than the biological properties and molecular biology of individual cell types that constitute developing target organs. Although the basic theory of hormone receptor action would apply to hormonal induction of macromolecular synthesis in individual cell types, it may be less applicable to more complex hormonal effects involving morphogenesis and cellular differentiation. In most of the systems studied so far, directive information between cells appears to proceed from mesenchyme toward epithelium, but communication in the reverse direction occurs in arteries from endothelium to smooth muscle[12] and in the kidney from the macula densa to the juxtaglomerular apparatus.[13]

During early pregnancy, the luminal epithelium performs a variety of functions that are essential for the eventual implantation of the blastocyst. Luminal epithelial cells maintain the metabolism of the blastocyst through the control of its intrauterine environment, provide an appropriate matrix for changes to occur at the interface between trophoblast and epithelium, and appear to transmit information from the blastocyst to the underlying stroma to initiate decidualization.[14] Our recent research has focused upon the mechanisms by which the luminal epithelium receives the signal of the blastocyst and transduces this stimulus into the initial uterine responses of implantation.

EPITHELIAL TRANSDUCTION OF A BLASTOCYST MESSAGE

Two of the earliest responses of the uterus to the presence of the blastocyst are changes in capillary permeability and signs of decidualization of stromal cells in the immediate vicinity of the blastocyst.[2,3] These responses could result from the direct effect of a chemical signal from the blastocyst upon endometrial stromal cells. Because the luminal epithelium appears intact during these responses, however, a direct effect would require the transmission of the signal through the epithelial layer. In the rabbit, prostaglandins (PGs) are able to transverse the uterine wall, but the uptake of PGs by epithelial cells probably involves dissolution into the lipid bilayer of cell membranes rather than binding to receptors or facilitated transport mechanisms.[15] Specific binding of PGE_2 to rat endometrial cell membrane preparations has been detected in stromal cells but not in luminal epithelial cells.[16,17]

Accumulated evidence suggests that luminal epithelial cells play a more active role in transmitting a message from the blastocyst to the stroma. When the luminal epithelium is experimentally removed from uterine horns sensitized by pretreatment with progesterone and estrogen, uteri become insensitive to both traumatic and nontraumatic deciduogenic stimuli.[14] Placement of a silk suture in the lumen of a sensitive uterus initiates a decidual reaction, but when this suture passes through only the serosa, myometrium, and stroma without reaching the luminal epithelium, no decidual reaction is observed.[18,19]

The transmission of the blastocyst message by the luminal epithelium to the stroma appears to require estrogen action. In ovariectomized pseudopregnant rats treated with only progesterone, initiation of decidualization requires a traumatic stimulus such as scratching or crushing, which damages the luminal epithelium.[20] If progesterone pretreatment is followed by estrogen, then non-traumatic stimuli will initiate decidualization.[2] Together these studies indicate that estrogen induces biochemical changes in the luminal epithelium which are prerequisites to blastocyst implantation in the rat.

If the transmission of a message from the blastocyst to underlying uterine tissues is one of the functions of epithelial cells, then the entire mechanism

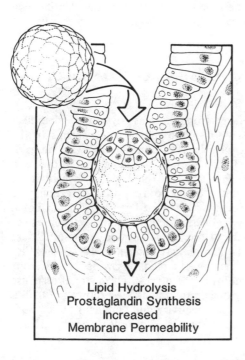

FIGURE 1. Possible response mechanism of luminal epithelial cells to the presence of the blastocyst.

Lipid Hydrolysis
Prostaglandin Synthesis
Increased
Membrane Permeability

of uterine sensitization becomes much more complex. Uterine sensitivity would require more than just the capacity of stromal cells and endometrial capillaries to respond to stimuli, physiologic or nonphysiologic, blastocyst or surgical trauma. Uterine sensitivity would also depend upon the capacity of epithelial cells to receive a message from the blastocyst and then to activate response mechanisms. These response mechanisms would then lead to the release of another message to underlying uterine tissues or perhaps the amplification of the original blastocyst message (FIG. 1).

Several candidates have been proposed over the years for the message sent from the blastocyst: a physical signal, histamine, estradiol, prostaglandins, and more recently, the catechol estrogens.[21,22] Various experiments over the years have shown that administration of these compounds will initiate events mimicking implantation and that inhibitors of their action will block implantation. Firm conclusions, however, have been difficult from these studies because of the complexities of the interrelationships between blastocyst, uterine tissues, and endocrine glands. Specificity and physiological relevance have been difficult to establish in such a complex system, which involves subtle mechanisms that can be easily overcome by nonspecific stimuli. For each of the above putative chemical messengers, there remains uncertainty concerning not only their source, but also their cellular targets. Identification of the message from the blastocyst would certainly be facilitated by the identification of very early and specific biochemical responses of specific uterine cells.

BIOCHEMICAL MECHANISMS OF MESSAGE TRANSDUCTION

On the other hand, if the message from the blastocyst were identified, then it would be much easier to establish the cellular mechanisms of the response to this signal—the biochemical basis of uterine sensitivity. Considerable physiologic and endocrine information is available that provides a framework for examining these mechanisms. Maximal uterine sensitivity is observed on day 5 if the day following proestrus during pseudopregnancy or the day that sperm is found during pregnancy is labeled day 1.[2,3] The hormonal requirements for uterine sensitivity in ovariectomized rats have been established: at least 36 hours of exposure to progestin followed by a small dose of estradiol. Maximum sensitivity is then observed some 12-18 h later (FIG. 2).[2,3] Submaximal decidualization can be obtained following progesterone treatment alone and traumatic stimulus of the uterus, but maximal response requires estradiol following progesterone pretreatment.[20] As shown in FIGURE 3, estradiol treatment increases uterine sensitivity and enhances the amount of decidual growth, but it also decreases the period of time during which the uterus is sensitive.[20]

Days	-2	-1	0	1	2	3	4	5	6	7
Pseudopregnancy	-	-	PE	-	-	-	-	sens.	-	-
Hormone treatment	E	E	-	-	MPA	-	e	sens.	-	-

PE = proestrus

E = 500ng estradiol

MPA = 3.5mg medroxyprogesterone acetate

e = 200ng estradiol

FIGURE 2. Uterine sensitivity during pseudopregnancy or following hormone treatment of ovariectomized rats.

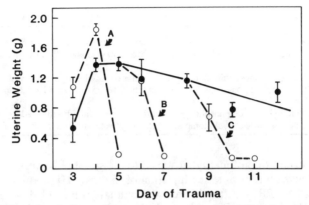

FIGURE 3. Effect of preliminary progesterone treatment on the ability of estrone and progesterone to promote deciduomal growth. Progesterone treatment (2 mg, ●----●), estrone and progesterone treatment (1 μg and 2 mg, ○----○). Curve A: estrone injections begun on day 1 with progesterone. Curve B: estrone injections begun on day 5 of progesterone treatment. Curve C: estrone injections begun on day 8 of progesterone treatment.[20]

With these hormonal and temporal data defining the system, there are several possible mechanisms by which the epithelial cells might respond to a signal from the blastocyst. The mechanisms listed in TABLE 1 are not mutually exclusive, but separately or together are means by which epithelial cells could receive a signal at the apical plasma membrane and respond with activation of enzyme pathways and with release of local chemical mediators. In these mechanisms the plasma membrane assumes great importance as the interface between uterus and blastocyst and as a source of arachidonic acid for PG synthesis. For a variety of cells, the transduction of signals acting on cell surface receptors appears to involve the methylation of membrane phospholipids.[23] The phospholipid methylation mechanism proposes that the methylation of membrane phospholipids increases membrane fluidity, which enhances the exposure or availability of hormone receptors and their coupling and activation of adenylate cyclases.[24] Features of the phospholipid methylation mechanism are diagrammed in FIGURE 4. Phospholipid methylation has been related to β-adrenergic receptor-adenylate cyclase coupling,[25] the mechanisms of action of several peptide hormones,[26–29] Ca^{2+}-dependent processes,[30] and chemotaxis.[31–33] We have examined the methylation of phospholipid for its involvement in the primary response of epithelial cells to the blastocyst.[34]

EPITHELIAL PHOSPHOLIPID METHYLATION AS A TRANSDUCING MECHANISM

Mature female rats were maintained and treated with progestin and estrogen following ovariectomy as previously described (FIG. 2). To determine

TABLE 1. Mechanisms for Transmission of Signals through Membranes

1. Adenylate cyclase activation, cAMP generation, activation of protein kinases.
2. Opening of membrane Ca^{2+} channels, Ca^{2+} influx, enzyme activation by calcium-calmodulin complexes.
3. Increased inositol phospholipid turnover, formation of diacylglycerol and inositol, 1,4,5-triphosphate, mobilization of calcium, protein kinase C activation, and arachidonic acid release (Nishizuka[23]).
4. Increased methylation of phospholipids, increased membrane fluidity, adenylate cyclase activation, calcium influx, arachidonic acid release (Hirata and Axelrod[24]).

in vivo incorporation of methyl groups into phospholipids, hormonally treated rats were given an intrauterine injection of [methyl-^{3}H] methionine (10 μCi/ horn in 25 μl PBS). After 15 min the animals were killed by cervical dislocation. Uteri were excised, trimmed of extraneous fat, and the lumen flushed with 3 ml of cold saline. Five uterine horns slit longitudinally were transferred to a round bottom tube containing 1 ml PBS and five 5 mm glass balls and mixed with a Vortex mixer for 2 min at 4°.[35] The epithelial cell fraction was removed with a Pasteur pipette, the remaining stroma-myometrium washed twice with 0.5 ml PBS, and the epithelial fraction homogenized once with a Polytron equipped with a PT10ST generator (Brinkmann Instruments, Westbury, N.Y.). The protein content of the epithelial fraction was determined,[36] and lipids were extracted with chloroform:methanol (2:1).[37,38] The organic phase was dried down under nitrogen at room temperature, redissolved in 25 μl of chloroform:methanol, and applied to an Anasil C thin layer plate. Phospholipid standards (phosphatidylethanolamine (PE), phosphatidylmon-

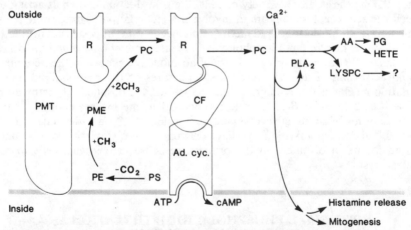

FIGURE 4. Coupling of phospholipid methylation to transmission of biological signals through cell membranes. Phospholipid methyltransferase (PMT); receptor (R); coupling factor (CF); adenylate cyclase (Ad. cyc.); phosphatidylserine (PS); phosphatidylethanolamine (PE); phosphatidyl-*N*-monomethylethanolamine (PME); phosphatidylcholine (PC); phospholipase A_2 (PLA$_2$); arachidonic acid (AA); prostaglandin (PG); 12-*L*-hydroxy-5,8,10,14-eicosatetraenoic acid (HETE); lysophosphatidylcholine (LYSPC).[24]

omethylethanolamine (PME), phosphatidyldimethylethanolamine (PMME), and phosphatidylcholine, (PC) 20 μg) were also applied to the plate, which was then developed with a solvent containing chloroform:propionic acid:n-propanol:water (3:2:6:1).[38] The location of lipids on the plate was determined with 0.2% dichlorofluorescein spray. One cm sections were scraped from the plate, suspended in 5 ml of Aquasol (New England Nuclear, Boston, Mass.), and the radioactivity was determined with a Packard Tri-Carb 460CD liquid scintillation counter (Packard, Downers Grove, Ill). *In vivo* incorporation of methyl groups into phospholipids was measured by determining the radio-activity in sections that corresponded to the cold PME, PMME, and PC standards.

FIGURE 5 shows changes in the capacity of uterine luminal epithelial cells to incorporate methyl groups into phospholipids during pseudopregnancy.

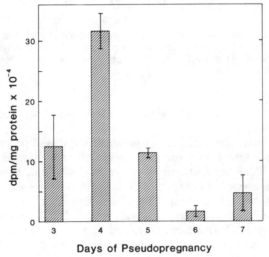

FIGURE 5. Effect of pseudopregnancy on the incorporation of ³H-methyl groups into epithelial phospholipid from [methyl-³H]methionine.[34]

Incorporation increased to maximal levels on day 4 of pseudopregnancy followed by decreases to low levels on days 6 and 7. The relative incorporation into PC decreased from 83% on day 4 to 62% on day 6. To examine the hormonal control of these changes, ovariectomized rats were treated as described in FIGURE 2 except that one group received the 200 ng injection of estradiol and the other did not. FIGURE 6 shows that levels of methylation of phospholipids in luminal epithelial cells decreased following estrogen treatment and that after 36 and 48 h of estradiol treatment, the level of incorporation was significantly less than after medroxyprogesterone acetate (MPA) treatment only ($p < 0.05$, t test). The relative incorporation into PC decreased from 55% to 40% after 36 h of estradiol treatment. In both of these experiments, levels of phospholipid methylation and the relative incorporation into

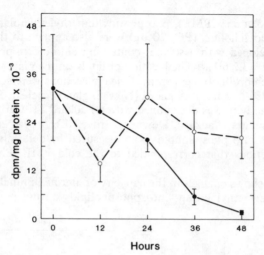

FIGURE 6. Effect of estradiol treatment of progestin-pretreated ovariectomized rats on the incorporation of ^{3}H-methyl groups into epithelial phospholipid from [methyl-^{3}H]methionine.[34] Ovariectomized rats were pretreated with medroxyprogesterone acetate for 48 h before treatment with estradiol (●) or vehicle (○).

PC decreased to lowest levels when the uterus had lost sensitivity to deciduogenic stimuli.

If phospholipid methylation is significantly involved in the transduction of deciduogenic stimuli that results in increased prostaglandin synthesis and increased capillary permeability as shown in FIGURE 7, then inhibition of this methylation would inhibit the increased capillary permeability following such a stimulus. Uterine phospholipid methylation can be inhibited by the intrauterine administration of 3-deazaadenosine (DZA, 13.3 μg/50 μl PO$_4$-buffered saline). DZA treatment decreased total incorporation into phospholipids by 80% and decreased the relative incorporation into PC from 55% to 36 percent. Ovariectomized rats were pretreated as shown in FIGURE 2 for sensitivity to a deciduogenic stimulus, and changes in capillary permeability were detected by measuring tissue concentrations of Evans blue, which infiltrates uterine tissue bound to plasma proteins. As shown in TABLE 2, treatment with DZA significantly inhibited the increase in capillary permeability following a deciduogenic stimulus.

During pseudopregnancy or following estrogen treatment of progestin-pretreated rats, the capacity of uterine epithelial cells to methylate phospholipids decreased to lowest levels when the uterus was no longer sensitive to deciduogenic stimuli. When phospholipid methylation was inhibited in luminal epithelial cells by DZA, uterine capacity for increases in vascular permeability following a deciduogenic stimulus was inhibited. These data suggest that responses of uterine luminal epithelial cells to deciduogenic stimuli may involve phospholipid methylation and that decreases in uterine sensitivity might result from decreases in cellular capacity for phospholipid methylation.

OTHER MECHANISMS AND STROMAL SENSITIVITY

As shown in TABLE 1, several of the cellular mechanisms for transmembrane transmission of signals involve the activation of adenylate cyclase and increased intracellular levels of adenosine $3'5'$ cyclic monophosphate (cAMP) as a second messenger. During early pseudopregnancy or following progesterone and estrogen treatment to induce uterine sensitivity, adenylate cyclase activity has been shown to increase to maximal levels at the time of uterine sensitivity.[39,40] Adenylate cyclase activity could be activated 2-5-fold by NaF treatment on all days of these treatments, but activation of the enzyme by uterine trauma was possible only at the time of uterine sensitivity (FIG. 8). Because the physicochemical properties of the uterine adenylate cyclase were not apparently altered by the endocrine status of the tissue, Yochim and his coworkers suggested that the transient capacity of the enzyme for activation in response to trauma might result from hormone-induced alterations of the membrane in which the adenylate cyclase was sequestered.[39,40]

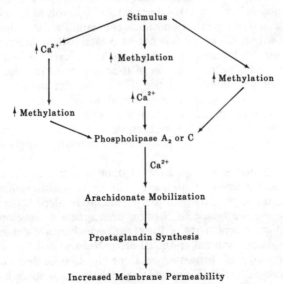

FIGURE 7. Potential relationships of calcium and phospholipid methylation to arachidonic acid mobilization and increased capillary membrane permeability.[53]

TABLE 2. Effect of 3-Deazaadenosine (DZA) on the Increase in Uterine Vascular Permeability in Response to a Deciduogenic Stimulus

Treatment[a]	Evans blue (μg/horn)		Ratio[b] Experimental:Control
	Experimental	Control	
PBSG	151.9 ± 12.8	64.8 ± 16.3	3.10 ± 0.54
PBSG + DZA	62.3 ± 11.5	68.6 ± 13.8	1.05 ± 0.24[c]

[a]Ovariectomized rats treated with estradiol and MPA as described in FIGURE 2 were given PBSG + DZA (33 μg/50 μl) or PBSG (50 μl) by transcervical injection of one uterine horn followed by two injections DZA (33 μg/20 μl PBS) or PBS (20 μl). Data are the mean ± SEM of eight rats.
[b]For each animal, the experimental horn to control horn ratio was calculated before the data were averaged.
[c]p < 0.01

Deciduogenic stimuli of sensitive uteri initiate rapid increases in uterine levels of cAMP[41-44] that can be inhibited by indomethacin, an inhibitor of prostaglandin synthesis.[43,44] Cholera toxin, a stimulator of adenylate cyclase, is also a potent inducer of endometrial vascular permeability changes in rats[44,45] and of decidualization in rats and mice.[43,44] From this evidence, it has been suggested that the involvement of prostaglandins in early decidualization may be mediated by changes in intracellular levels of cAMP.[21] For many cell types, PGEs increase adenylate cyclase activity, and many of the biological effects of the PGEs are thought to be mediated by activation of this system complex.[46] Although activation of adenylate cyclase and increased intracellular levels of cAMP appear to be involved in uterine sensitization and the early response to deciduogenic stimuli, the cellular location of these events within the uterus has not been established. Adenylate cyclase activation within the luminal epithelium could indicate an involvement of this enzyme in epithelial transduction of the message of the blastocyst. Activation of the enzyme complex in the cells of the endometrial stroma, the vascular endothelium or stroma cells, would suggest a mechanism for responses of these tissues to PGs and a basis for uterine sensitization. As pointed out later, binding sites for PGs have been detected only in stromal cells,[16,17] and uterine levels of these binding sites increase following progesterone treatment.[16]

Although this discussion has focused upon changes in uterine luminal epithelial cells as the basis for uterine sensitivity to deciduogenic stimuli, it would be a mistake to presume that uterine sensitivity depends entirely upon biochemical changes in these cells. Stromal cells appear to develop a capacity for decidualization, a sensitivity of their own, which is not dependent upon a message from intact luminal epithelial cells. Nonsensitive uteri of ovariectomized rats treated with progesterone alone can initiate decidualization in response to traumatic stimuli that damage the luminal epithelium.[20] Nontraumatic stimuli such as intrauterine oil or phosphate-buffered saline containing gelatin (PBSG) do not initiate decidualization and yet stimulate increases in vascular permeability[47] and in tissue levels of PG.[48] Clearly, nonsensitized uteri respond to nontraumatic stimuli and with responses that are usually considered integral components of decidualization. Perhaps the responses are of insufficient strength or duration to initiate decidualization. Milligan and Mirembe offer possible explanations for the failure of nonsensitive uteri to respond fully with decidualization to nontraumatic stimuli.[47] If permeability changes and decidualization each depend upon different uterine signals, then sensitivity following estrogen treatment could depend upon uterine capacity to produce another signal along the lines of our previous discussion. Another possibility is that decidualization depends upon development of the capacity of stromal cells to respond to a signal from the epithelium.

Stromal sensitivity to deciduogenic stimuli could result from a reprogramming of the cellular capacities of endometrial stromal cells, the acquisition of PG binding sites, for example, during cell cycles prior to blastocyst implantation. In several cellular systems, altered gene activity for cell differentiation requires prior DNA synthesis.[49] During the day prior to uterine sensitivity, populations of endometrial stromal cells synthesize DNA and undergo a round of mitosis. These events are controlled by progesterone and estradiol.[4] In ovariectomized rats hormonally treated for sensitivity to deciduogenic stimuli, both progestin and estradiol treatment stimulated DNA synthesis in endometrial stomal cells that later differentiated into deciduomal

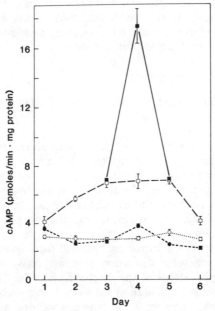

FIGURE 8. Effect of progesterone and estrone on uterine adenylate of cyclase activity in pseudopregnant rats ovariectomized on day 2. ○----○, vehicle control; ●----●, progesterone, 2 mg; □--- ---□ progesterone, 2 mg + estrone, 1 μg; ■----■, progesterone + estrone + trauma.[40]

cells.[50] Coincident with endometrial DNA synthesis and mitosis during early pseudopregnancy, levels of binding sites for PGs increased in the uterine endometrium.[51] Progesterone pretreatment of ovariectomized rats increased levels of binding sites for PGs that were not increased by further treatment with estradiol to yield uterine sensitivity to nontraumatic stimuli.[16] PG binding sites were detected only in membrane preparations from stromal cells after progesterone treatment.[16] Stromal acquisition of these PG binding sites could explain the sensitization of these cells to traumatic deciduogenic stimuli.

Since stromal growth and differentiation following a deciduogenic stimulus requires increased gene expression with the initiation of active RNA synthesis, the development and loss of uterine sensitivity to deciduogenic stimuli could result from changes in uterine chromatin template activity. Uterine chromatin template activity was measured following progesterone and progesterone plus estradiol treatment by determining the number of initiation sites available for RNA transcription.[52] As uteri of ovariectomized rats attained sensitivity following progesterone treatment, the number of RNA initiation sites increased 5-fold. Termination of uterine sensitivity by sequential estradiol treatment as described earlier (FIG. 3) depressed the transcriptive activity of uterine chromatin below control levels within 4 h, although the uterus remained fully sensitive for another 26 hours. Because the loss of uterine chromatin template activity was more rapid following estradiol treatment than after simple progesterone withdrawal, it appeared that estradiol actively restricted template activity. Although the cellular location of changes in template capacity has not been identified, it seems reasonable that these effects of progesterone and estradiol indicate another mechanism functioning in endometrial stromal cells to control sensitivity to deciduogenic stimuli.

SUMMARY AND CONCLUSIONS

In our discussion of responses of the uterine epithelium to the blastocyst and their relationship to sensitization to deciduogenic stimuli, we have attempted to identify pieces of information that could be arranged into possible mechanisms. These choices and the limits of space resulted in a great deal of information that was not mentioned: changes in the charge and composition of the glycocalyx of the luminal epithelium, the morphology of the apical surface of the epithelium, steroid hormone receptor levels, epithelial protein synthesis, and most of the information obtained from species other than rats and mice. Despite whatever distortion that may have resulted from our reductions and simplifications of the mechanisms of implantation, it should be clear that blastocyst implantation involves communication not only between blastocyst and uterus, but also between various uterine tissues. Our understanding of implantation will be improved if we can identify the responses of individual tissues and the mechanisms of this communication. It seems likely that development and loss of uterine sensitivity controlled by progesterone and estradiol will depend upon separate biochemical responses in specific uterine tissues.

ACKNOWLEDGMENTS

We would like to thank Marcia Hartsock for the illustrations and Vickie Stidham for the careful preparation of the manuscript.

REFERENCES

1. SHELESNYAK, M. C. 1957. Some experimental studies on the mechanism of ovaimplantation in the rat. Recent Prog. Horm. Res. **13**: 269-322.
2. FINN, C. A. 1977. The implantation reaction. *In* Biology of the Uterus. R. M. Wynn, Ed. 245-308. Plenum Press. New York.
3. PSYCHOYOS, A. 1973. Endocrine control of egg-implantation. *In* Handbook of Physiology, Endocrinology. R.O. Greep & E.B. Astwood, Eds. Vol. 2 (part 2): 187-215. Am. Physiological Society. Washington, D.C.
4. HEALD, P. J. 1976. Biochemical aspects of implantation. J. Reprod. Fertil. (Suppl) **25**: 29-52.
5. QUARMBY, V. E. & L. MARTIN. 1982. Qualitative effects of progesterone on estrogen binding in mouse uterine luminal epithelium. Mol. Cell. Endocrinol. **27**: 331-342.
6. MAIRESSE, N. & P. GALAND. 1982. Estrogen-induced proteins in luminal epithelium, endometrial stroma and myometrium on the rat uterus. Mol. Cell. Endocrinol. **28**: 671-679.
7. MOULTON, B. C. & B. B. KOENIG. 1983. Progestin increases cathepsin D synthesis in uterine luminal epithelial cells. Am. J. Physiol. **244**: E442-E446.
8. QUARMBY, V. E. & K. S. KORACH. 1984. Differential regulation of protein synthesis by estradiol in uterine component tissues. Endocrinology **115**: 687-697.
9. WILCE, P. A., L. LEIJTEN & L. MARTIN. 1984. Stimulation of 3-hydroxy-3-methylglutaryl-coenzyme A reductase in mouse uterine epithelial cells by oestradiol-17 beta. Biochem. J. **218**: 849-855.
10. LEJEUNE, B., F. LAMY, R. LECOCQ, J. DESCHACHT & F. LEROY. 1985. Patterns of protein synthesis in endometrial tissues from ovariectomized rats treated with oestradiol and progesterone. J. Reprod. Fertil. **73**: 223-228.
11. CUNHA, G. R., L. W. K. CHUNG, J. M. SHANNON, O. TAGUCHI & H. FUJII. 1983. Hormone-induced morphogenesis and growth: Role of mesenchymal-epithelial interactions. Recent Prog. Horm. Res. **39**: 559-598.
12. FURCHGOTT, R. F. 1983. Role of endothelium in responses of vascular smooth muscle. Circ. Res. **53**: 557-573.
13. NAVAR, L. G. & L. ROSIVALL. 1984. Contribution of the renin-angiotensin system to the control of intrarenal hemodynamics. Kidney Int. **25**: 857-868.
14. LEJEUNE, B., J. VAN HOECK & F. LEROY. 1981. Transmitter role of the luminal uterine epithelium in the induction of decidualization in rats. J. Reprod. Fertil. **61**: 235-240.
15. CAO, Z.-D., M. A. JONES & M. J. K. HARPER. 1984. Prostaglandin translocation from the lumen of the rabbit uterus *in vitro* in relation to day of pregnancy or pseudopregnancy. Biol. Repord. **31**: 505-519.
16. KENNEDY, T. G., D. MARTEL & A. PSYCHOYOS. 1983. Endometrial prostaglandin E_2 binding during the estrous cycle and its hormonal control in ovariectomized rats. Biol. Reprod. **29**: 565-571.

17. JONES, M. A. & M. J. K. HARPER. 1983. Prostaglandin accumulation by isolated uterine endometrial epithelial cells from six-day pregnant rabbits. Biol. Reprod. **29:** 1201-1209.
18. FAINSTAT, T. 1963. Extracellular studies of uterus. I. Disappearance of the discrete collagen bundles in endometrial stroma during various reproductive states in the rat. Am. J. Anat. **112:** 337-350.
19. LEJEUNE, B. & F. LEROY. 1980. Role of the uterine epithelium in inducing the decidual cell reaction. *In* Progress in Reproductive Biology. F. Leroy, C. A. Finn, A. Psychoyos & P. O. Hubinont, Eds. Vol. **7:** 92-101. S. Karger. Basel, Switzerland.
20. YOCHIM, J. M. & V. J. DE FEO. 1963. Hormonal control of the onset, magnitude and duration of uterine sensitivity in the rat by steroid hormones of the ovary. Endocrinology **72:** 317-326.
21. KENNEDY, T. G. 1983. Embryonic signals and the initiation of blastocyst implantation. Aust. J. Biol. Sci. **36:** 531-543.
22. MONDSCHEIN, J., R. M. HERSEY, S. K. DEY, D. L. DAVIS & J. WEISS. 1985. Catechol estrogen formation by pig blastocysts during the preimplantation period: Biochemical characterization of estrogen-2/4-hydroxylase and correlation with aromatase activity. Endocrinology. **117:** 2339-2346.
23. NISHIZUKA, Y. 1984. Turnover of inositol phospholipids and signal transduction. Science **225:** 1365-1370.
24. HIRATA, F. & J. AXELROD. 1980. Phospholipid methylation and biological signal transmission. Science **209:** 1082-1090.
25. HIRATA, F., W. J. STRITTMATTER & J. AXELROD. 1979. Beta-adrenergic receptor agonists increase phospholipid methylation membrane fluidity and beta-adrenergic receptor-adenylate cyclase coupling. Proc. Natl. Acad. Sci. USA **76:** 368-372.
26. BHATTACHARYA, A. & B. K. VONDERHAAR. 1979. Phospholipid methylation stimulates lactogenic binding in mouse mammary gland membranes. Proc. Natl. Acad. Sci. USA **76:** 4489-4492.
27. MILVAE, R. A., H. W. ALILA & W. HANSEL. 1983. Methylation in bovine luteal cells as a regulator of luteinizing hormone action. Biol. Reprod. **29:** 849-855.
28. NIETO, A. & K. J. CATT. 1983. Hormonal activation of phospholipid methyltransferase in the Leydig cell. Endocrinology **113:** 758-762.
29. KELLY, K. L., F. L. KIECHLE & L. JARETT. 1984. Insulin stimulation of phospholipid methylation in isolated rat adipocyte plasma membranes. Proc. Natl. Acad. Sci. USA **81:** 1089-1092.
30. CREWS, F. T., Y. MORITA, A. MCGIVENY, F. HIRATA, R. P. SIRAGANIAN & J. AXELROD. 1981. IgE-mediated histamine release in rat basophilic leukemia cells: Receptor activation, phospholipid methylation, Ca^{2+} flux and release of arachidonic acid. Arch. Biochem. Biophys. **212:** 561-571.
31. HIRATA, F., B. A. CORCORAN, K. VENKATASUBRAMANIAN, E. SCHIFFMAN & J. AXELROD. 1979. Chemoattractants stimulate degradation of methylated phospholipids and release of arachidonic acid in rabbit leukocytes. Proc. Natl. Acad. Sci. USA **76:** 2640-2643.
32. PIKE, M. C., N. M. KREDICH & R. SNYDERMAN. 1979. Phospholipid methylation in macrophages is inhibited by chemotactic factors. Proc. Natl. Acad. Sci. USA **76:** 2922-2926.
33. MATO, J. M. & D. MARIN-CAO. 1979. Protein and phospholipid methylation during chemotaxis in *Dyctostelium discoideum* and its relationship to calcium movements. Proc. Natl. Acad. Sci. USA **76:** 6106-6109.
34. MOULTON, B. C. & B. B. KOENIG. 1986. Hormonal control of phospholipid methylation in uterine luminal epithelial cells during sensitivity to deciduogenic stimuli. Endocrinology. **118:** 244-249.
35. FAGG, B., L. MARTIN, L. ROGERS, B. CLARK & V. E. QUARMBY. 1979. A simple method for removing the luminal epithelium of the mouse uterus for biochemical studies. J. Reprod. Fertil. **57:** 335-339.
36. LOWRY, O. H., N. J. ROSEBROUGH, A. L. FARR & R. J. RANDALL. 1951. Protein measurement with folin phenol reagent. J. Biol. Chem. **193:** 265-275.
37. KATES, M. 1972. Techniques of lipidology. Isolation, Analysis and Identification of Lipids. 351-353. Am. Elsevier Publishing Company. New York.

38. HOOK, V. Y. H., S. HEISLER & J. AXELROD. 1982. Corticotropin-releasing factor stimulates phospholipid methylation and corticotropin secretion in mouse pituitary tumor cells. Proc. Natl. Acad. Sci. USA **79:** 6220-6224.

39. BEKAIRI, A. M., R. B. SANDERS & J. M. YOCHIM. 1984. Uterine adenylate cyclase activity during the estrous cycle and early progestation in the rat: Responses to fluoride activation and decidual induction. Biol. Reprod. **31:** 742-751.

40. BEKAIRI, A. M., R. B. SANDERS, F. S. ABULABAN & J. M. YOCHIM. 1984. Role of ovarian steroid hormones in the regulation of adenylate cyclase during early progestation. Biol. Reprod. **31:** 752-758.

41. LEROY, F., J. VANSANDE, G. SHETGEN & D. BRASSEUR. 1974. Cyclic AMP and the triggering of the decidual reaction. J. Reprod. Fertil. **39:** 207-211.

42. RANKIN, J. C., B. E. LEDFORD & B. BAGGETT. 1977. Early involvement of cyclic nucleotides in the artificially stimulated decidual cell reaction of the mouse uterus. Biol. Reprod. **17:** 549-554.

43. RANKIN, J. C., B. E. LEDFORD, H. T. JONSSON & B. BAGGETT. 1979. Prostaglandins, indomethacin and decidual cell reaction in the mouse uterus. Biol. Reprod. **20:** 399-404.

44. KENNEDY, T. G. 1983. Prostaglandin E_2, adenosine 3':5'-cyclic monophosphate and changes in endometrial vascular permeability in rat uteri sensitized for the decidual cell reaction. Biol. Reprod. **29:** 1069-1076.

45. JOHNSTON, M. E. A. & T. G. KENNEDY. 1984. Estrogen and uterine sensitization for decidual cell reaction in the rat: Role of prostaglandin E_2 and adenosine 3':5'-cyclic monophosphate. Biol. Reprod. **31:** 959-966.

46. SAMUELSSON, B., E. GRANSTROM, K. GREEN, M. HAMBERG & S. HAMMARSTROM. 1975. Prostaglandins. Annu. Rev. Biochem. **44:** 669-695.

47. MILLIGAN, S. R. & F. M. MIREMBE. 1985. Intraluminally injected oil induces changes in vascular permeability in the 'sensitized' and 'non-sensitized' uterus of the mouse. J. Reprod. Fertil. **74:** 95-104.

48. MILLIGAN, S. R. & F. D. C. LYTTON. 1983. Changes in prostaglandin levels in the sensitized and non-sensitized uterus of the mouse after the intrauterine installation of oil or saline. J. Reprod. Fertil. **67:** 373-377.

49. MACLEAN, N. 1977. The Differentiation of Cells. 49-58. University Press. Baltimore, Md.

50. MOULTON, B. C. & B. B. KOENIG. 1984. Uterine deoxyribonucleic acid synthesis during preimplantation in precursors of stromal cell differentiation during decidualization. Endocrinology **115:** 1302-1307.

51. KENNEDY, T. G., M. DOMINIQUE & A. PSYCHOYOS. 1983. Endometrial prostaglandin E_2 binding: Characterization in rats sensitized for the decidual cell reaction and changes during pseudopregnancy. Biol. Reprod. **29:** 556-564.

52. GLASSER, S. R. & S. A. McCORMACK. 1979. Estrogen-modulated uterine gene transcription in relation to decidualization. Endocrinology **104:** 1112-1118.

53. CRAVEN P. A. & F. R. DERUBERTIS. 1984. Phospholipid methylation in the calcium-dependent release of arachidonate for prostaglandin synthesis in renal medulla. J. Lab. Clin. Med. **104:** 480-493.

Endocytosis in the Rat Uterine Epithelium at Implantation[a]

MARGARET B. PARR AND EARL L. PARR

Department of Anatomy
School of Medicine
Southern Illinois University
Carbondale, Illinois 62901

INTRODUCTION

Endocytosis is a striking feature of luminal epithelial cells in uteri of rats and mice during the peri-implantation period.[1-5] Tracers such as ferritin, horseradish peroxidase, or Thorotrast introduced into the uterine lumen were rapidly incorporated into vacuoles up to 3 μm in diameter formed by apical protrusions, or pinopods, and into small, coated, pinocytotic vesicles (0.1 μm). Thereafter, the material taken into the epithelial cells by endocytosis was channeled into lysosomes. Initially, the lysosomes containing the tracer were restricted to the apical halves of the epithelial cells, but they soon moved throughout the cells.[6] Such movement was dependent on microtubules, because colchicine treatment blocked the migration of lysosomes to the basal halves of the cells.[7,8]

Lysosomes containing tracer were often seen near the basolateral membranes, but no exocytosis of tracer into the intercellular spaces or basal stroma was observed by light or electron microscopy either in animals during early pregnancy, in ovariectomized rats treated with hormones, or during delayed implantation. This contrasts with reports that trypan blue was transported into the stroma after uterine trauma, or in animals given daily injections of progesterone and estrogen.[2] Enders and Nelson[3] reported that rats on day 5 of gestation and in delayed implantation that had ferritin in the uterine lumen for 1 hr or longer showed small tubules containing ferritin in the peripheral cytoplasm and extracellularly in the lateral and basal aspects of the intercellular spaces. Also, horseradish peroxidase was observed in an occasional intercellular space following prolonged exposure to the tracer. The authors point out that massive amounts of protein placed in the lumen are not physiological and that some of the uteri exposed for 60 min or longer showed

[a]This work was supported by NIH research Grant HD 17480.

dilation of the outer cellular spaces beyond the normal variation for the stage examined. Further studies are needed to determine whether material taken up at the apical surface can be transported across the cell and released into the extracellular spaces.

The distribution of uterine cells that take up tracers or display pinopods is irregular. With scanning electron microscopy the lining of the uterine lumen showed areas free of projections, isolated individual pinopods, or pinopods arranged in clusters and rows.[3,9,10] More cells of the antimesometrial side of the uterus, the site of implantation, showed pinopods and took up trypan blue and ferritin than those at the mesometrial side, both on day 5 of pregnancy and during delayed implantation in the rat.[1,6] These preliminary observations deserve closer study. There did not appear to be any differences in the distribution of endocytotic cells along the length of the uterine horns, and pinopods were observed adjacent to unimplanted blastocysts and in inter-implantation sites.

Apical endocytosis in the uterus is under ovarian hormone control and was observed only during progestational periods. In the rat, the uptake of trypan blue occurred on days 5 and 6 of pregnancy, during pseudopregnancy, and at the site of local progesterone injection, but not during the estrous cycle or after ovariectomy.[1,11] Other tracers such as ferritin were shown to be endocytosed by uterine epithelial cells during early pregnancy, with a distinct peak of activity on day 5 in the rat[3,4,6] and day 4 in the mouse.[5] A day later in each case there was a marked decrease in the number of cells containing tracer molecules. Treatment of ovariectomized rats with proges-terone alone, or with estradiol followed by progesterone, caused uptake of intraluminally administered trypan blue and ferritin, whereas estradiol alone did not cause the same.[12] Endocytosis of ferritin also occurred during lac-tational delayed implantation[3] and during delayed implantation obtained by ovariectomy during early pregnancy followed by daily injections of proges-terone in the rat[10] and the mouse.[5] The administration of nidatory estradiol to animals in delayed implantation had no effect on endocytosis 24 hrs later, but after 48 hrs the endocytosis had ceased (unpublished observations[5]).

The function of apical endocytosis in the peri-implantation period remains unknown. Although selective uptake of materials cannot be excluded it seems likely that pinopods mediate bulk uptake of macromolecules from the lumen, which are hydrolyzed in secondary lysosomes. Digestion products could then diffuse back into the uterine lumen to alter the molecular environment of the blastocysts, or they could pass to the underlying stroma to provide an indirect mechanism for transferring information from the lumen to the stroma. Direct transepithelial passage of macromolecules from the uterine lumen into the stroma may[2,3] or may not[6,12] occur. The reasons for these differences are not clear, and the fate of luminal material taken into the uterus by endocytosis is worth further study.

In addition to possible functions already suggested,[3,4,12] endocytosis may be part of a process that regulates implantation by controlling the properties of the epithelial cell apical membrane. The fate of membrane that is internalized by endocytosis is not yet fully understood, but numerous studies have demonstrated that endocytosis is coupled to exocytosis or secretion in a variety of cells (for references see 6). Thus, as surface membrane is taken in by endocytosis, it is replaced by secretory vesicle membrane. Electron microscopic images of rat uterine epithelial cells on day 5 of pregnancy suggested the secretion of a class of electron-transparent vesicles.[13,14] The vesicles appeared to originate from the Golgi complex, accumulate in the apical part of the cell, and fuse with the apical surface membrane at the base of the microvilli. Several other observations are consistent with this view. The vesicles developed and disappeared in conjunction with endocytosis, but did not take up ferritin. A similarity of the vesicle and apical membrane was suggested by periodic acid-silver proteinate staining. In addition, the apical vesicles and Golgi cisternae were normally located in the apical halves of the epithelial cells, and both were shifted together to the basal portions of the cells by colchicine treatment, providing further evidence that the apical vesicles were derived from the Golgi complex.[8,13] Endocytosis and its coupled exocytosis may maintain the apical membrane of epithelial cells in a preparatory condition for implantation. This is consistent with the occurrence of endocytosis on days 4 and 5 of pregnancy and throughout delayed implantation. After the estrogen secretion on day 4 of pregnancy or after estrogen administration to animals in delayed implantation, endocytosis gradually decreases, the properties of the apical membrane may change, and implantation can proceed.

In addition to endocytosis at the apical surface of uterine epithelial cells during early pregnancy, endocytosis of intravenously injected horseradish peroxidase has been demonstrated at the basolateral membranes.[14,15] The endocytotic vesicles combined with intracellular tubular or irregularly shaped vesicles that then moved across the cell towards the luminal surface. There, electron microscopic images suggested they may fuse with the apical membrane to release their contents into the uterine lumen by exocytosis. Thus, there appears to be transepithelial movement of horseradish peroxidase from base to apex. Furthermore, there may be a role for basolateral endocytosis in the implantation process because this activity increased 4- to 5-fold during the early implantation period, and in ovariectomized animals treated with an ovarian hormonal regimen that prepares the uterus for implantation. These observations suggest that there is intracellular transepithelial movement of macromolecules from the blood and/or stroma into the uterine lumen. Because the direct passage of substances between the intercellular spaces and the uterine lumen is blocked by tight junctions,[16] which are particularly deep and complex during the implantation period,[17] the intracellular pathway may account for the presence of macromolecules such as plasma proteins in the uterine fluid.[18] The transported macromolecules may be required for endometrial sterility, protection of the blastocyst against immunological rejection, or blastocyst implantation and development.

The purpose of the present investigation was to study further the pinocytotic activity at the basolateral membranes of uterine epithelial cells during the implantation period by following the uptake of fluorescein-labeled bovine serum albumin (BSA), immunoglobulin G (IgG), and apoferritin administered intravenously.

MATERIAL AND METHODS

Virgin female Holtzman rats (Sasco, Inc., Omaha, Nebraska) 60 to 100 days old, maintained under a light program of 12L:12D, were used in these experiments. The animals were mated and the day on which spermatozoa were found in the vaginal smear was designated day 1 of pregnancy. On days 6 and 7 of pregnancy the rats were anesthetized with tribromoethanol, and 0.5 ml of 1% pontamine sky blue dissolved in saline was injected into the femoral vein. Immediately thereafter 50 mg of fluorescein isothiocyanate (FITC)-labeled bovine serum albumin (BSA), bovine immunoglobulin G (IgG), or apoferritin dissolved in 1 ml saline was administered to the rat using the opposite femoral vein. One rat on day 7 was given 120 mg of labeled IgG in 1 ml saline. After 10 min, 30 min, 1, 4, 5, or 7 hr, the rats were killed, and the uterine horns were removed from the animals, cut into segments containing implantation sites and interimplantation regions, and fixed by immersion in 10% formalin in 0.1 M sodium phosphate buffer, pH 7.4 (4°C) for 24 hours. Three rats on day 7 were each given 0.8 mg of free fluorescein, approximating the amount of FITC conjugated to 120 mg of IgG. These rats were killed after 10 min, 1 hr, and 4 hr, and their uteri were processed as above. The fixed tissues were washed in buffer, dehydrated, and embedded in polyethyleneglycol 1000 (PEG) according to the method of Masurkiewicz and Nakane (1972). Uteri were sectioned at 6 μm and mounted on polylysine-coated slides (Wolosewick and De Mey, 1982). The PEG was removed from the sections by sequential treatment with limonene and absolute alcohol. The sections were dried and mounted in a mixture of 50% ethanol, 45% glycerol, and 5% phosphate-buffered saline (PBS). Coverslips were then sealed to the slides with clear nailpolish to minimize evaporation of the mounting medium. Uterine sections from 82 implantation sites and numerous nonimplantation sites from 30 rats were examined with a Nikon or Olympus fluorescence microscope. In two rats on day 7 of pregnancy, the right oviduct was cut at the uterotubual junction before BSA or IgG was administered intravenously; the animals were killed 4 or 5 hr later. One to four rats were used at each time point for each tracer, and at least two implantation sites were examined from each rat.

Immunoglobulin G and apoferritin were conjugated to FITC using the method of Goding (1976). Fluorescein-conjugated BSA was purchased from Sigma Chemical Co., St. Louis, Missouri. The molar fluorescein/protein ratios, measured essentially as described by Thé and Feltkamp[19] were: BSA, 2.5; IgG, 5.0; and apoferritin, 15.

RESULTS

In general, at implantation sites on days 6 and 7 of pregnancy, intravenously administered FITC-labeled BSA, IgG, and apoferritin were located

TABLE 1. Localization of FITC-Labeled Proteins in Rat Uterine Epithelia

		Fluorescence Observed			
		Implantation site		Inter-implantation site	
Tracer and day of pregnancy	Time after administration	LE[a]	GE	LE	GE
Day 6					
BSA	10 min	−[b]	−	−	−
	30 min	−	+ +	−	−
	1 hr	+ +	+ +	+ +	−
	5 hr	+ +	+ +	+	+
Apoferritin	4 hr	+ +	+ +	+	+
Day 7					
BSA	10 min	−	−	−	−
	30 min	+	+	−	−
	1 hr	+	+	+ +	−
	5 hr	+ +	+ +	+ +	+
	7 hr	−	+	−	−
IgG	1 hr	−	−	+	−
	4 hr	+[c]	+	+	−
	7 hr	+[c]	−	+	−
Apoferritin	7 hr	+ +	+ +	+	+

[a]LE = luminal epithelium; GE = glandular epithelium.
[b]− = no fluorescence in epithelial cells; + = fluorescence present in some epithelial cells; + + = fluorescence present in most epithelial cells.
[c]Fluorescence was present only in the transitional epithelium.

in maternal blood vessels, luminal and glandular epithelial cells, and in the uterine lumen. At interimplantation sites, there was fluorescence in maternal vessels, but none or relatively little at the other locations. Tracer fluorescence was never observed in gland lumina, nor was it observed anywhere in the uterine horns of rats injected with free fluorescein for 10 min, 1 hr, or 4 hours. Our observations on the uptake of FITC-labeled proteins into luminal and glandular epithelia are summarized in TABLE 1.

At implantation sites on days 6 and 7 of pregnancy there was little or no tracer fluorescence in epthelial cells at 10 or 30 min after administration of FITC-BSA. At these times there was fluorescence in the basement membrane and in the intercellular spaces of the epithelia up to the region of the tight junctions (FIG. 1a). At 60 min there were small, uniform-sized fluorescent

FIGURE 1a-c. a. Photomicrograph of luminal epithelial cells from the implantation site of a rat on day 6 of pregnancy 10 min after receiving FITC-BSA. Note the fluorescence in the stromal spaces, along the basement membrane and in the intercellular spaces of the luminal epithelium (arrows). b. Luminal epithelial cells at the implantation site from a rat on day 7 of pregnancy 1 hr after receiving FITC-BSA. Fluorescence is present in the sites mentioned in FIGURE 1a and in small uniform-sized granules (arrow) throughout the cells. c. Glandular epithelial cells from a rat on day 6 of pregnancy 1 hr after receiving FITC-BSA. Fluorescence is present in small granules (arrow); a, b, and c × 330.

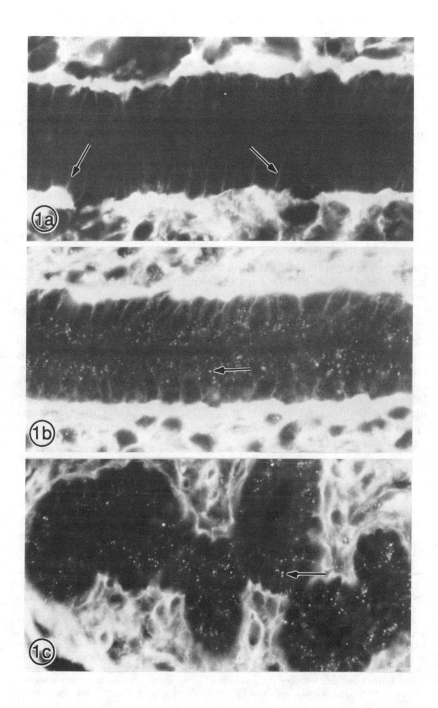

granules in some glandular and luminal epithelial cells (FIGS. 1b and 1c). At 5 hr there was fluorescence in small granules in most epithelial cells and often in the uterine lumen or along the apical borders of the luminal epithelial cells (FIGS. 2a, 2b, and 2c). In some sites fluorescence was also observed in large, uniform-sized granules, 2-3 μm in diameter and in the apical halves of cuboidal transitional epithelial cells located between the ectoplacental cone and the columnar cells at the mesometrial side of the uterus (FIGS. 2b and 2c). There was also fluorescence in the uterine cavity adjacent to these epithelial cells.

In implantation sites at 1, 4, or 7 hr after administration of 50 mg of FITC-IgG, little or no tracer was present in the small, uniform granules in epithelial cells. Tracer was present in the uterine lumen at 4 and 7 hr, and also in the large granules in the apical halves of transitional epithelial cells (FIG. 3a), as seen after injection of labeled BSA. In one rat that received 120 mg of FITC-IgG for 4 hr, fluorescence was observed as above and also in the small, uniform-sized granules in some luminal epithelial cells. The distribution of labeled BSA and IgG in the uteri of rats whose uterotubal junctions were transected before treatment was similar to that in intact animals, indicating that little, if any, tracer entered the uterine lumen from the oviduct.

In implantation sites at 4 or 7 hr after the administration of FITC-labeled apoferritin, fluorescent granules were present in the luminal epithelium but showed regional variation. In five sites from four rats there were small, uniform-sized granules in the epithelium at the mesometrial side of the uterus, similar to those seen using BSA as tracer, whereas the transitional epithelium toward the antimesometrial side was free of tracer. In three implantation sites from four rats there were fluorescent granules of variable size in the mesometrial epithelium and granules of small, uniform size in the transitional epithelium (FIG. 3b). In all cases the glandular epithelium contained small, uniform granules (FIG. 3c).

SUMMARY AND DISCUSSION

In these studies we describe the localization of intravenously administered FITC-labeled BSA, IgG, and apoferritin in implantation and interimplan-

---

FIGURES 2a-c. These micrographs were taken from the same histological section. They show the uterine lumen and luminal epithelial cells from an implantation site of a rat uterus on day 7 of pregnancy 5 hr after the administration of FITC-BSA. **a.** Mesometrial epithelial cells are columnar and show fluorescence in small faint granules. There is no tracer fluorescence in the uterine lumen; $\times$ 440. **b.** This is a region antimesometrial to that shown in FIGURE 2a. Note the fluorescence in the uterine lumen (arrowhead) and in larger granules (arrow) located primarily in the apical halves of the epithelial cells that are cuboidal in this region (transitional epithelium); $\times$ 330. **c.** Transitional region adjacent to that seen in 2b showing fluorescence in the uterine lumen (arrowhead) and in larger granules (arrow) in the apical portions of the epithelial cells. Note that fluorescent granules are limited to those cells adjacent to tracer in the uterine lumen; $\times$ 330.

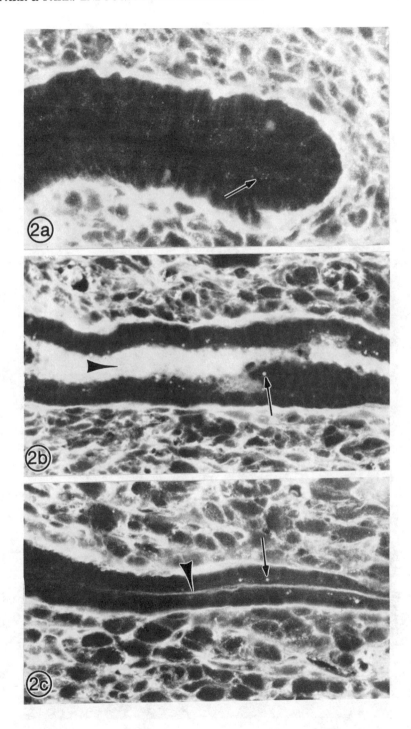

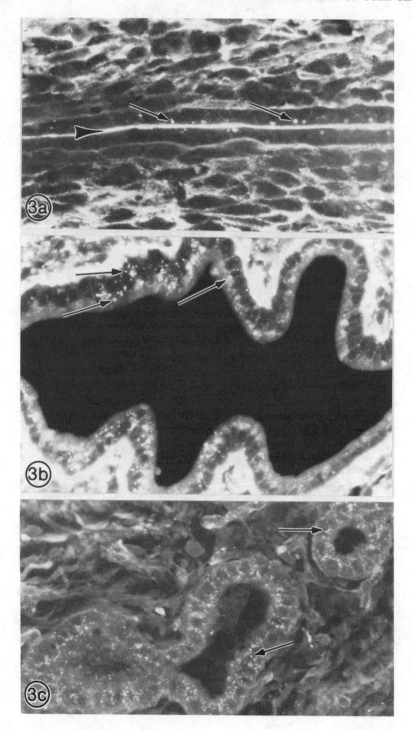

tation sites of rat uteri on days 6 and 7 of pregnancy. We believe that the fluorescein observed in the tissues was bound to intact tracer proteins because no specific fluorescence was present in the uterus at 10 min, 1 hr, or 4 hr after administration of free fluorescein. It appeared that unconjugated fluorescein was not fixed in the tissue by the histological procedures used for these studies.

At implantation sites, tracer fluorescence was observed in small, uniform-sized granules in at least some luminal and glandular epithelial cells at 1 and 5 hr after administration of labeled BSA, at 4 hr after injection of 120 mg of IgG, and at 4 and 7 hr after treatment with labeled apoferritin. All three tracers were observed in the uterine lumen at the longer time points, especially in the transitional region between the ectoplacental cone of the embryo and the columnar epithelium at the mesometrial side of the uterus. No fluorescence was detected in the gland lumina. Labeled BSA and IgG were observed in large granules, 2-3 μm in diameter, in the apical part of the cuboidal epithelial cells in the transitional region and in the adjacent uterine lumen. We did not detect the large fluorescent granules in transitional epithelial cells using apoferritin as a tracer. In several implantation sites from the apoferritin-treated rats, however, columnar epithelial cells at the mesometrial side of the uterus that were not in contact with tracer protein in the uterine lumen contained fluorescent granules of variable size. This may suggest a different intracellular fate for this protein, as compared to BSA and IgG, which were found only in small, uniform-sized granules in the mesometrial epithelium. At interimplantation sites the epithelial cells lacked fluorescence or showed a smaller number of the small fluorescent granules; tracer fluorescence was not detected in the uterine lumen.

The presence of tracer fluorescence in the uterine lumen at implantation sites after administration of all three labeled proteins indicates that plasma proteins do reach the uterine lumen at this time. Tracer proteins did not enter the uterine lumen from the oviduct in large amounts, if at all, because they were present in the uterine lumina of rats whose uterotubal junctions had been transected. The pathway for the passage of tracer proteins into the uterine lumen is not known. The transport may be intracellular and follow a pathway similar to that described for horseradish peroxidase on day 5 of pregnancy in rats.[14] We suggest that the uptake of FITC-labeled proteins from plasma into small, uniform granules in both luminal and glandular epithelia may be due to the activity of such a transepithelial transport process. The release of such proteins into the uterine lumen has not been demonstrated,

---

FIGURE 3a-c. **a.** Transitional epithelial cells from a rat 4 hr after being injected with FITC-IgG on day 7 of pregnancy. Fluorescence is located in the uterine lumen (arrowhead) and in large granules (arrows) in the apical parts of the cuboidal epithelium; × 330. **b.** Luminal epithelial cells at the mesometrial side of the uterus from a rat 7 hr after being injected with FITC-apoferritin on day 7 of pregnancy. Note fluorescence in small and large granules (arrows). There is no tracer fluorescence in the adjacent uterine lumen; × 290. **c.** Glandular epithelial cells from a rat 4 hr after the administration of FITC-apoferritin on day 6 of pregnancy showing fluorescence in small granules (arrows); × 400.

however. If such transport occurs, it is surprising that the tracer proteins were not observed in gland lumina, and it is not clear why the tracer proteins in the uterine lumen were particularly abundant adjacent to the transitional epithelium. It is possible that plasma proteins pass into the uterine lumen between epithelial cells in the transitional region. These cells are morphologically distinct at this stage because they have changed from columnar to cuboidal, and they will progressively degenerate during the next few days as the placenta develops.[20] By days 6 and 7 of pregnancy their intercellular junctions may be leaky, thus allowing plasma proteins to pass into the uterine lumen and accumulate in the transitional region.

The presence of large fluorescent granules in the apical part of transitional epithelial cells adjacent to labeled BSA and IgG in the uterine lumen may indicate the uptake of these tracers from the uterine lumen. Using immunohistochemical techniques, Rachman et al.[21] have demonstrated IgG in the uterine lumen and in large granules in the epithelium at the comparable time and location in mice; they, too, suggested that the transitional epithelium was probably taking up protein from the lumen. The significance of the presence of serum proteins at this site awaits further studies.

ACKNOWLEDGMENTS

We thank Kimberly Munaretto, Robin Sigler, and Bruce Jones for their excellent technical assistance and Candida Trueblood for typing the manuscript.

REFERENCES

1. VOKAER, E. 1952. Recherches histophysiologiques sur l'endométre du rat, en particulier sur le conditionnement hormonal de ses propriétes athrocytaires. Arch. Biol. Liège **63:** 1-84.
2. SARTOR, P. 1969. Athrocytose du bleu trypan par l'endométre de la ratte. Manifestation du processus en fonction du contexte hormonal. C.R. Acad. Sci. **163:** 2564-2567.
3. ENDERS, A. C. & D. M. NELSON. 1973. Pinocytotic activity of the uterus of the rat. Am. J. Anat. **138:** 277-300.
4. PARR, M. B. & E. L. PARR. 1974. Uterine luminal epithelium: protrusions mediate endocytosis, not apocrine section, in the rat. Biol. Reprod. **11:** 220-233.
5. PARR, M. B. & E. L. PARR. 1977. Endocytosis in the uterine epithelium in the mouse. J. Reprod. Fertil. **50:** 151-153.
6. PARR, M. B. & E. L. PARR. 1978. Uptake and fate of ferritin in the uterine epithelium of the rat during early pregnancy. J. Reprod. Fertil. **52:** 183-188.
7. PARR, M. B., M. G. KAY & E. L. PARR. 1978. Colchicine inhibition of lysosome movement in the rat uterine epithelium. Cytobiologie **18:** 374-378.
8. PARR, M. 1979. A morphometric analysis of microtubules in relation to the inhibition of lysosome movement caused by colchicine. Eur. J. Cell Biol. **20:** 189-194.

9. PSYCHOYOS, A. & P. MANDON. 1971. Etude de la surface de l'epithelium uterin au microscope electronique a bayalage. Observations la Ratte au 4ᵉ et au 5ᵉ jour la gestation. C.R. Acad. Sci. Ser. D 272: 2723-2725.

10. PARR, M. B. 1983. Relationship of uterine closure to ovarian hormones and endocytosis in the rat. J. Reprod. Fertil. 68: 185-188.

11. VOKAER, R. & F. LEROY. 1962. Experimental study on local factors in the process of ova implantation in the rat. Am. J. Obstet. Gynecol. 83: 141-148.

12. LEROY, F., J. VAN HOECK & C. BOGAERT. 1976. Hormonal control of pinocytosis in the uterine epithelium of the rat. J. Reprod. Fertil. 57: 49-62.

13. PARR, M. B. 1982. Apical vesicles in the rat uterine epithelium during early pregnancy: A morphometric study. Biol. Reprod. 26: 915-924.

14. PARR, M. B. 1980. Endocytosis at the basal and lateral membranes of rat uterine epithelial cells during early pregnancy. J. Reprod. Fertil. 60: 95-99.

15. PARR, M. B. 1982. Effects of ovarian hormones on endocytosis at the basal membranes of rat uterine epithelial cells. Biol. Reprod. 26: 909-913.

16. ANDERSON, W., Y. KANG & E. DE SOMBRE. 1975. Endogenous peroxidase: specific marker enzyme for tissue displaying growth dependancy on estrogen. J. Cell Biol. 64: 668-681.

17. MURPHY, C. R., J. G. SWIFT, T. M. MUKHERJEE & A. W. ROGERS. 1982. The structure of tight junctions between uterine luminal epithelial cells at different stages of pregnancy in the rat. Cell Tissue Res. 223: 281-286.

18. SURANI, M. A. H. 1977. Qualitative and quantitative examination of the proteins of rat uterine luminal fluid during pro-oestrus and pregnancy and comparison with those of serum. J. Reprod. Fertil. 50: 281-287.

19. THÉ, T. H. & T. E. W. FELTKAMP. 1970. Conjugation of fluorescein isothiocyanate to antibodies. 1. Experiments on the conditions of conjugation. Immunology 18: 865.

20. KREHBIEL, R. H. 1937. Cytological studies of the decidual reaction during pregnancy and in the production of deciduomata. Physiol. Zool. 10: 212-238.

21. RACHMAN, F., V. CASIMIRI & O. BERNARD. 1984. Maternal immunoglobulins G, A, & M in mouse uterus and embryo during the postimplantation period. J. Reprod. Immunol. 6: 39-47.

Progesterone Action in Preparation for Decidualization[a]

J. M. YOCHIM

Department of Physiology and Cell Biology
University of Kansas
Lawrence, KS 66045, USA

INTRODUCTION

During the early stages of gestation, the uterine milieu becomes transformed from an environment hostile to the presence of the conceptus to one that actively supports the process of nidation and pregnancy. This transformation requires the action of progesterone in almost all mammals studied. Though we have learned much about the changing morphologic and functional character of the uterus during these early progestational stages, we know very little of the specific actions of progesterone that induce the differentiational changes. Research during the past quarter century has revealed many puzzling characteristics about this hormone, questions that still remain unanswered: What function does the initial "priming" by estrogen serve in a uterus whose metabolism, once primed, is subsequently inhibited by actions of progestogen? Why is there a requirement for so much progestogen relative to the level of estrogen during the initiation and maintenance of progestation? How does estrogen augment progestogen action in the face of a progestogenic blockade of almost every major effect of estrogen? What key aspects of metabolism, controlled by progestogen, define this hormone's ability to induce the changes required for implantation and pregnancy? How is this metabolism altered following the stimulus to induce decidualization?

None of these questions can be answered adequately at the present time. Indeed, though research has refined and redefined the questions, the answers remain elusive. What I propose during this short presentation is to describe the results of studies done by several groups, not just ours, in a context that may provide some insight to these problems. Whether or not these ideas are correct will obviously require verification through more experimentation. I believe, however, that they are worth considering, and this symposium, in honor of Professor Shelesnyak, provides an excellent forum for such an endeavor.

[a] This work was supported in part by University of Kansas General Research Fund Grant #3971 and Biomed Grant #4171.

122

ORDERS OF MAGNITUDE

FIGURE 1 shows a general relationship between the plasma concentrations of estradiol and progesterone in the pseudopregnant rat, and the Kd of these hormones for their uterine receptors. If we assume that there is an unimpaired diffusion of the hormones into the uterine cells, it becomes apparent that simple relationships among plasma levels, intracellular receptor binding, and biological activity are difficult to construct.

For example, because the plasma estrogen level appears too low (10^{-11} - 10^{-10} M) to generate a significant rise on the saturation curve, we should see

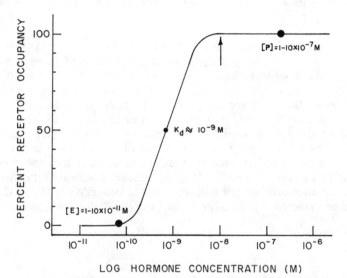

LOG HORMONE CONCENTRATION (M)

FIGURE 1. General relationship between the approximate equilibrium dissociation constants (Kd) of uterine estradiol and progesterone receptors and the plasma molar concentrations of these hormones (E,P) during pseudopregnancy in the rat. The arrow indicates the uterine receptor occupancy if the plasma levels of progesterone were reduced by 95%.

minimal receptor-dependent biologic activity.[1,2] Yet, in the rat the actions of the hormone at this level are essential during early progestation; at higher or lower concentrations, progestation may be impaired.

By contrast, the plasma progesterone concentration (10^{-7} - 10^{-6} M) is well beyond intracellular receptor saturation.[1,3,4] Theoretically, a decrease in the hormone's plasma level by as much as 95% (arrow, FIG. 1) should not impair maximum receptor binding. Because this hypothetical plasma concentration of progesterone (10^{-8} M) would still be at least 10-fold greater than the Kd for its receptor, receptor-dependent biological activity should remain high. This simple calculation raises a curious question: Of what biological significance is the "excess" progesterone, if its only destiny is to be metabolized and excreted?

Indeed, if our hypothetically decreased plasma progesterone concentration does not affect receptor binding (FIG. 1), it may well reduce the amount of hormone metabolized by the uterus, and it must be noted that such a decrease in the hormone level can impair progestation.[5-7] Thus, there appears to be a bonafide requirement for high concentrations of progesterone to maintain normal progestation. To examine this problem it is worthwhile to review a few aspects of the metabolism of progesterone by the target cell.

HOW IS PROGESTERONE METABOLICALLY INACTIVATED?

In the uterus of the rat, most studies reveal that between 25-35% of the end products of progesterone metabolism are a result of 5α-reductase activity.[8-11] Additional metabolic reduction of the steroid is achieved by other NADP-dependent enzymes as well.[11] Consequently, high plasma and target tissue levels of this hormone can generate an appreciable amount of reduced product,[12] and such activity may induce a measurable drain on the NADP-dependent reductive machinery of the uterine cell, thus altering uterine metabolism. The evidence suggests that aspects of progesterone action may be dependent not only on hormone-receptor interaction, but upon the hormone's inactivation by way of specific NADP-dependent systems. With this background, we may examine one such response to progestogen: the modulation of pyridine nucleotide metabolism related to NADP synthesis, as depicted in FIGURE 2.[13,14]

HOW DO THE OVARIAN STEROIDS REGULATE NAD METABOLISM?

A major effect of estrogen in this system (FIG. 2) is its ability to induce the synthesis of estrogen and progesterone receptors.[15] It is here that the important priming effects of estrogen are manifested. Yet, during progestation, such activity may be transient and time-dependent, because as progesterone levels increase during early progestation, this action of estrogen may be indirectly modulated. Indeed, in some systems there is evidence that progesterone may limit its own ability to act in the uterus by way of a hormone-receptor mechanism.[15-19]

A second effect of estrogen shown in FIGURE 2 is the induction of NAD-glycohydrolase (NAD-GH).[20-22] The cytoplasmic (microsomal) form of the enzyme may support the adenosine diphosphate (ADP)-ribosylation of various cytoplasmic or membrane proteins, whereas the NAM is recycled by way of a salvage path to resynthesize NAD. The nuclear enzyme can act as a poly(ADP-ribosyl) transferase. In both the rat and mouse, estrogen priming increases the activity of uterine nuclear NAD-glycohydrolase (FIG. 2, 3A).[20,22] Inhibition of estrogen-induced activity through this pathway by NAM, a product inhibitor of the enzyme, prevents the incorporation of thymidine into DNA.[20] Thus, these actions of estrogen may be important in regulating DNA synthesis, but they tend to decrease the availability of NAD for NADP synthesis.

A third action of estrogen is the induction of a steroid 5α-reductase in the uterine nucleus.[10,11] After about three days of estrogen stimulation in the

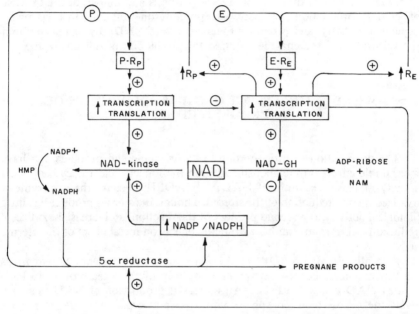

FIGURE 2. Comparison of receptor-mediated actions of progesterone on NAD metabolism with actions resulting from the metabolic reduction of progesterone. R_P, R_E = progesterone, estrogen receptors; NAD = nicotinamide adenine dinucleotide; NADP = nicotinamide adenine dinucleotide phosphate; NAM = nicotinamide; HMP = hexose monophosphate pathway; NAD-GH = NAD-glycohydrolase.

rat, this nuclear enzyme shows significant activity that persists even in the presence of progesterone. Similarly, the activity of this enzyme, high in the endometrium during the preovulatory period, also shows measurable activity at the time that sensitivity to decidualization is imminent.[12] By contrast, an extranuclear 5α-reductase in uterine cells is not sensitive to estrogen.[11] Both the nuclear and cytoplasmic enzymes require NADPH as a coenzyme.

Progesterone increases the activity of NAD-kinase, the enzyme required for NADP synthesis (FIG. 2, 3B).[23] The hormone also increases the concentration of NAD and blocks an estrogen-induced increase in NAD-glycohydrolase activity (FIG. 3A).[21,22,24,25] Estrogen has little effect on NAD-kinase activity, and does not seem to interfere with the stimulatory action of progesterone on NAD-kinase. These actions of progesterone tend to shift metabolism to favor NADP synthesis by increasing both the substrate and the enzyme. The shift may serve to favor cell differentiation, but it may also inhibit DNA synthesis and cell division, as described below.

The evidence thus indicates that as part of its priming effect, estrogen augments both the ability of progesterone to interact with its receptor and the ability of the cell nucleus to metabolize progesterone by way of a reductive pathway. Both effects may be transient and ultimately suppressed by subsequent actions of progesterone. In addition, the hormone stimulates aspects of NAD metabolism that support DNA synthesis and mitosis at the expense of NADP production. By contrast, progesterone inhibits this estrogen-dependent activity, and promotes the synthesis of NADP by increasing both the substrate and the enzyme required for production of this coenzyme.

WHAT IS THE EFFECT OF THE 5α-REDUCTION OF PROGESTERONE?

The degradation of progesterone to its pregnane end products can have measurable effects on metabolism. In both the nucleus and the cytosol, such activity increases the ratio of $NADP^+/NADPH$, because the coenzyme is oxidized during reduction of the steroid. Though the steroid product has little biological activity, the second product of the reaction, an increased oxidized/reduced NADP ratio, can have dramatic effects on metabolism of the uterine cell.

A locally elevated $NADP^+/NADPH$ ratio in extranuclear compartments permits an increased NADP synthesis by way of the release of a blockade against NAD-kinase (FIG. 2).[26] An increased production of NADP can activate the hexose monophosphate path, to produce pentoses, and to recycle the oxidized NADP to its reduced form. Both products are required for reductive biosynthetic activity. In the nucleus, an elevated $NADP^+$ induced by the estrogen-sensitive reductase may inhibit ADP-ribosylation of nuclear protein.[27] Such activity can alter the rate of estrogen-induced DNA synthesis.

Accordingly, with the more than tenfold rise in progesterone levels during early progestation, the metabolic reduction of this hormone would be increased to a rate that is limited only by the availability of the reduced coenzyme, NADPH. Such action can occur during days 3-5 of progestation in the rat, but later, this activity may be reduced, because the progestogen, through its generally inhibitory actions, may depress the synthesis of the estrogen-dependent 5α reductase.[8,9] The cytoplasmic reductase activity may not be so affected.

Thus, the active degradation of progesterone by the steroid reductase can provide an $NADP^+/NADPH$ ratio that, in the nucleus, may delay or decrease the rate of DNA synthesis, and in the cytoplasm, favors production of more $NADP^+$ and activation of the hexose monophosphate path. These actions, a result of the metabolism of progesterone, appear to augment similar effects of the hormone manifested through classical hormone-receptor interactions (see FIG. 2).

HOW IS NAD METABOLISM RELATED TO PROGESTATION?

During progestation in the rat, or under hormone regimes in which progesterone is dominant, NAD, NADP, and NAD-kinase increase, whereas

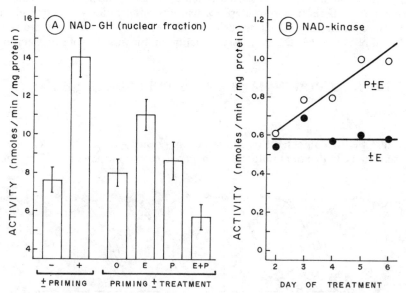

FIGURE 3. Effect of estrone and progesterone on (A) NAD-glycohydrolase (NAD-GH)[22] and (B) NAD-kinase activity in the endometrium of the rat.[23] Ovariectomized animals were primed with estrone (5.0 μg/day) for 3 days and rested for 1 day prior to daily replacement therapy beginning on day 1 of the experiment. NAD-GH was measured on day 4, whereas NAD-kinase was measured during days 2-6. E = 1.0 μg estrone/day; P = 2.0 mg progesterone/day; N = 6 rats per point.

NAD-GH activity decreases.[22–24,28,29] The stimulation of the NAD-kinase pathway by progesterone can be correlated with an increased NADP concentration, and the maintenance of RNA synthesis and cell differentiation. The inhibition of the GH pathway by progesterone can be correlated with the elevated NAD concentration, a reduced polyADP-ribosylation of chromatin protein, and with a subsequently decreased rate of DNA synthesis and mitosis in the progestional uterus.

For example, examination of the endometrium of the rat during early progestation reveals that as the level of progesterone rises, epithelial mitoses are blocked and the rate of stromal mitosis is retarded compared with the equivalent stages of the estrous cycle (FIG. 4).[30] Similarly, in an *in vitro* system, progesterone can delay the cell cycle in endometrial cells of the rabbit.[31]

A pyridine nucleotide metabolite (NAM) that can block the activity of NAD-GH can simulate this phenomenon, altering the sensitivity to decidual induction in the rat. If NAM is injected during the wave of stromal cell division that precedes the onset of uterine sensitivity, then sensitivity is inhibited; if NAM is administered following this wave of stromal mitosis, then sensitivity is augmented somewhat (FIG. 5).[32]

Thus, the NAM-induced blockade that inhibits sensitivity (FIG. 5) probably removes cohorts of cells from a cell cycle and mitosis that is required prior to the differentiation to uterine sensitivity; after mitosis, injection of the vitamin encourages postmitotic cell differentiation by increasing the availability of NAD for NADP synthesis, an action mimicking that of progesterone.

DOES ESTROGEN HAVE A DOSE-DEPENDENT, BIPHASIC ACTION?

It is well documented that in the rat (and other species) the development of sensitivity to decidual induction is dependent on an interaction of estrogen

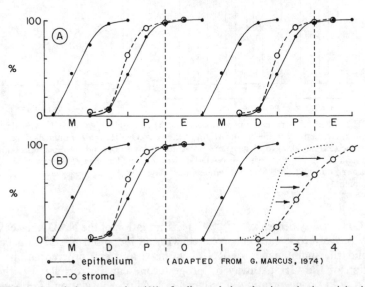

FIGURE 4. Cumulative proportion (%) of cell population showing mitotic activity in endometrium during the estrous cycle (A) and during early progestation (B). During days 2-3 of progestation, there occurs an inhibition of epithelial mitoses and a delay in stromal mitoses (arrows) compared with that during the estrous cycle (dotted line). P = proestrus; E = estrus; M = metestrus; D = diestrus. Recalculated from data of Marcus.[30]

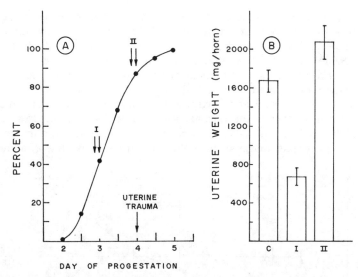

FIGURE 5. Effect of nicotinamide (NAM) on sensitivity of the uterus to decidual induction. A: Cumulative proportion of stromal cell population undergoing mitosis during early pseudopregnancy, adapted from Marcus.[30] Shown at I and II are the times of injection of NAM in each of two groups of rats. Each group was traumatized at 1200 h day 4 to induce decidualization. B: Response of the uterus on day 9 to an intraluminal decidual-inducing stimulus at 1200 h day 4; adapted from Yochim.[32] C = control; 100 mg NAM was injected i.p. at 0900 and 1200 h on day 3 (group I) or on day 4 (group II).

with progestogen. It is equally well known that an estrogen-deficient, progestogen-maintained uterus can respond to strong traumatic stimuli, albeit in a limited fashion. By contrast, the estrogen-stimulated, progestogen-deficient uterus is unresponsive to traumatic stimuli. Such experiments reveal that it is the progestogen that is necessary for the development of uterine sensitivity to decidual induction; the estrogen can augment or inhibit sensitivity in the rat, but it cannot induce it (FIG. 6).[5,33]

With this background, let us consider the experimental animal primed with estrogen, but maintained with only progesterone for several days. Based on hormone-receptor interaction, the response of the uterus to estrogen-priming would include, among many other parameters, an increase in synthesis of progesterone receptors. Those aspects of progesterone action that require hormone-receptor interaction may be supported, including the synthesis of NAD-kinase, and the inhibition of many estrogen-induced anabolic responses.

By day 4 of progestogen treatment, the estrogen-deprived uterus is unable to provide adequate machinery for extensive estrogen-dependent anabolic activity, but it can still metabolize progesterone by way of several cytoplasmic NADP-dependent enzymes that do not require maintenance by estrogen. Two major shifts in extranuclear NAD metabolism may occur as a result of the increased $NADP^+/NADPH$ ratio: an inhibition of NAD-GH activity and a release from inhibition of NAD-kinase activity.

Both changes contribute in different ways (increased enzyme activity, increased substrate) to an augmentation of NADP production by way of the NAD-kinase pathway. As a result, the concentration and content of endometrial NADP are increased dramatically in the progesterone-maintained, estrogen-deprived uterus, and cytoplasmic metabolic responses that support differentiation are favored.[29]

Note that though nuclear 5α-reductase activity is probably not maintained in this animal, neither is the estrogen-sensitive nuclear glycohydrolase (see FIG. 3). Thus, DNA synthesis would proceed at a slow, but uninhibited rate. Under the prevailing marginal anabolic conditions, those few endometrial

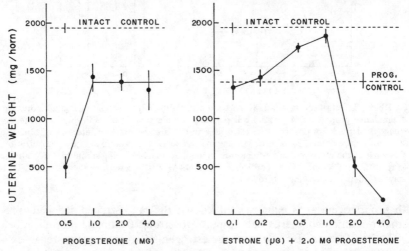

FIGURE 6. Effect of estrone and progesterone on uterine sensitivity to decidual induction. Rats were ovariectomized on day 1 of pseudopregnancy and treated with progesterone ± estrone during days 1-3. Following traumatization on day 4, animals were injected daily until day 9 with 1.0 μg estrone + 2.0 mg progesterone to support decidual growth. The results, measured as uterine weight ± SE on day 9, reflect the hormone treatments administered during days 1-3.[33]

stromal cells that have undergone a recent mitosis can differentiate and will respond to traumatic stimuli in a manner that is absolutely dependent on the level of progesterone to which the cells have been exposed (FIG. 6).[33,34] This metabolic model may simulate the conditions that exist during a lactationally delayed implantation in the rat.

If "permissive" levels of estrogen are introduced into this system, the intranuclear metabolism of progesterone may be maintained. Activity of the nuclear 5α reductase metabolizes progesterone and oxidizes NADPH. These local changes can serve to block any nuclear glycohydrolase activity that may have been augmented by this low-level estrogen (FIG. 3). As a result, DNA synthesis would still be retarded. At this level of estrogen, however, some cytoplasmic anabolic activity is also augmented (increased oxidative metabolism and rate of protein synthesis).[35,36] This activity may contribute to a more effective program of differentiation induced by the progestogen-stimulated rise in NADP synthesis. The response of the uterus to a decidual stimulus will be augmented over that in the estrogen-deprived animal (FIG. 6).[33]

Finally, with high estrogen levels imposed on the system, more of the effects of progesterone are damped. An estrogen-induced increase in glycohydrolase activity within both the nuclear and cytoplasmic compartments may shift NAD metabolism and reduce the availability of substrate for NADP synthesis. ADP-ribose production increases, and though many more cells can now be recruited into the mitotic cell cycle, fewer can undergo a postmitotic differentiation, owing to the relatively depressed rate of NADP formation. The uterus will be less responsive to decidual stimuli (FIG. 6).[33]

Thus, low levels of estrogen, insufficient to promote uterine growth, nonetheless can maintain sufficient anabolic activity to augment progestogen-induced differentiation. High levels of estrogen reduce the progestogen-induced shift in NAD metabolism, thus promoting uterine growth and mitosis at the expense of progestational differentiation.

HOW IS METABOLISM ALTERED BY A DECIDUAL STIMULUS?

If the preparation of the uterus of the rat for implantation requires a modulation of pyridine nucleotide metabolism that supports differentiation, then the induction of the decidual response requires the opposite, a metabolism that permits almost unrestricted growth: DNA synthesis, mitosis, hyperplasia, and hypertrophy. How can the metabolism of a progesterone-dominated tissue be altered so rapidly by an external signal? How can such changes be wrought in the presence of the high plasma levels of progestogen required to maintain pregnancy? Indeed, is progesterone required for this action?

Though the mechanism by which the decidual stimulus is transduced is not clearly defined, the result of that transduction has been shown to alter a key aspect of pyridine nucleotide metabolism. Within 30 minutes following the application of a traumatic stimulus to uteri maintained by progestogen, NAD-kinase activity is dramatically inhibited (FIG. 7).[23] The inhibition can be demonstrated in uteri treated with progesterone or with progesterone/estrogen combinations, but not in endometria maintained with estrogen alone. Clearly, the response requires the prior action of progesterone.

Effectively, the trauma to the uterus reduces the NADP synthesizing capacity of the endometrium by about 60-80%, thereby reducing the general availability of the coenzyme. Though such a decline may increase the availability of NAD in only a minor way, it may have several significant indirect effects on NAD-GH activity.

A reduction in NADP synthesis (by way of inhibition of NAD-kinase) effectively decreases the absolute levels of $NADP^+$. As a result, the block against NAD-GH may be relieved. In addition, the inability of the NADPH-dependent 5α-reductase machinery to operate at pretrauma levels (owing to a decline in the coenzyme) may further reduce this blockade, because the extensive oxidation of NADPH is decreased. In the nucleus, an inhibition of poly(ADP-ribosyl) transferase may be relieved, allowing an increase in the rate of DNA synthesis. Thus, the tissue metabolism may be altered to support decidual growth.

It is of some significance that the inhibition of NAD-kinase activity by uterine trauma is not a temporally delimited phenomenon. Strong stimuli, applied after the period of uterine sensitivity are as effective in inhibiting the

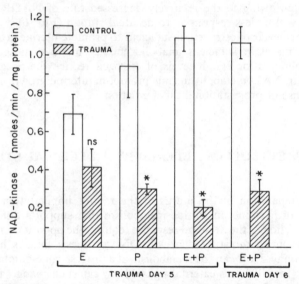

FIGURE 7. Effect of trauma to the uterus on endometrial NAD-kinase activity in ovariecto-mized, hormone-maintained rats.[23] Following estrogen priming (5.0 μg estrone/day) for 3 days, and 1 day rest, animals were treated with estrone (E, 1.0 μg/day), progesterone (P, 2.0 mg/day) or the combination of hormones. In this system, deciduomata cannot be induced after day 5 in animals treated with E+P. ns = no significant difference in enzyme activity between control and traumatized horns; * = difference in activity between control and traumatized horns significant at p < 0.05; n = 3 experiments/point.

enzyme as those administered during the time of sensitivity (FIG. 7).[23] The evidence indicates that the inhibition of NAD-kinase activity is dependent on a prior progestogenic action, but is independent of those estrogen-sensitive factors that regulate the duration of sensitivity to decidual induction.

Furthermore, because the activity of NAD-kinase can be altered without inducing decidual growth, it is obvious that the two processes are not tightly coupled; rapid inhibition of the progestogen-dependent enzyme activity by uterine trauma is not a stimulus for the onset of progestogen-dependent decidual growth following the trauma. Though deciduogenesis may require the shift in pyridine nucleotide metabolism, such metabolic changes act only to support, not to initiate, decidual growth.

The data indicate that we may consider the activity of the progestogen-sensitive NAD-kinase pathway to be of key importance in the metabolism of the preimplantation progestational uterus. Its inhibition following a decidual-inducing stimulus is a modulation of this metabolic activity consistent with the onset of growth of the decidua.

HOW DOES THE DECIDUAL STIMULUS ALTER METABOLISM?

The properties of NAD-kinase provide a number of intriguing clues that may link the enzyme to the transduction of the decidual stimulus.[14] Because the transduction mechanisms have not yet been clearly defined, it is possible only to speculate, without much evidence, but it may be worthwhile to submit one such idea for consideration.

A role for the adenylate cyclase system as part of the transducing mechanism for the decidual stimulus has been suggested by several investigators.[37-40] The activity of this enzyme in the uterus of the rat is controlled by estrogen and progestogen in a fashion different from the roles of these hormones in the regulation of sensitivity to decidual induction. Whereas uterine sensitivity is a progestogen-dependent phenomenon, augmented and temporally limited by low levels of estrogen, adenylate cyclase is an estrogen-sensitive enzyme whose baseline activity is not affected by progestogen.[33,40]

Nonetheless, like sensitivity to decidual induction, this enzyme can be activated dramatically by gentle trauma to the uterus, but only on day 4 of progestation.[39] The response (and its transient nature) requires a uterus that has been exposed to both estrogen and progestogen, and the activation itself is evidenced within 30 seconds following such a trauma (FIG. 8).[40,41] This response may be among the initial events leading to decidual induction.

The intriguing links between adenylate cyclase and NAD metabolism are that (a) the activation of adenylate cyclase may require an increased glyco-hydrolase activity for ADP-ribosylation of the regulatory subunit of the cyclase enzyme and (b) the product of the activated cyclase, cAMP, is an inhibitor of NAD-kinase activity.[42-44] Thus, in this system, the trauma may activate estrogen-dependent systems (NAD-GH and adenylate cyclase) that can ultimately lead to inhibition of a progestogen-dependent system (NAD-kinase). Because the latter response permits a further rise in glycohydrolase activity, a positive feedback cascade may be initiated.

Whether or not a cause-effect relationship exists between the activation of uterine adenylate cyclase and the subsequent inhibition of NAD-kinase remains to be investigated. Indeed, before such a relationship can be demonstrated, one bit of contradictory evidence, based on timing, will require resolution: though NAD-kinase activity can be inhibited by trauma applied 24 hours after the period of uterine sensitivity (FIG. 7), the rapid activation of adenylate cyclase by trauma is limited to the period of maximal sensitivity to decidual induction.[23,39,40] Thus, it is possible to induce an inhibition of NAD-kinase activity without activating adenylate cyclase or inducing a decidual response.

SUMMARY

An attempt has been made to describe several actions of progesterone related to the preparation of the uterus for decidualization. These actions result from classical ligand-receptor interactions as well as from nonreceptor-mediated changes, that is, those imposed by metabolic inactivation of the

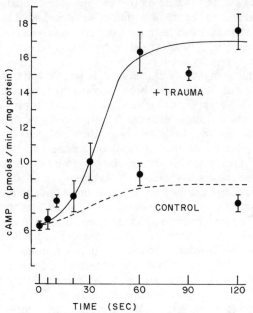

FIGURE 8. Time course of adenylate cyclase activation following a mild trauma to the uterus on day 4 of pseudopregnancy. Values are the means ± SEM for 3-4 rats/point.[41]

steroid. By opposing some of the effects of estrogen, the progestogen alters the utilization of NAD in the endometrium to induce an increase in $NADP^+$ production, elevation of the $NADP^+/NADPH$ ratio, and inhibition of the rate of degradation of NAD to NAM and ADP-ribose. These changes are correlated with (a) an inhibition or delay in endometrial DNA synthesis and mitosis, (b) an increased potential for differentiation, and (c) the development of uterine sensitivity to decidual induction. A decidual-inducing stimulus can reverse these progestogen-dependent effects rapidly by limiting the rate of synthesis of $NADP^+$ from NAD. Though one possible mechanism for this reversal may include the inhibition of NAD-kinase by cAMP, there is evidence to suggest that such a direct cause-effect relationship is at present tenuous.

REFERENCES

1. BUTCHER, R. L., W. E. COLLINS & N. W. FUGO. 1975. Endocrinology **96:** 576.
2. SMITH, M. S., M. E. FREEMAN & J. D. NEILL. 1975. Endocrinology **96:** 219.
3. CHEESMAN, K. L. & R. T. CHATTERTON JR. 1982. Endocrinology **111:** 564.
4. PEPE, G. J. & I. ROTHCHILD. 1974. Endocrinology **95:** 275.
5. DE FEO, V. J. 1967. *In* Cellular Biology of the Uterus. R. M. Wynn, Ed.: 191. Appleton Century Crofts. New York.
6. RAZIANO, J., M. FERIN & R. L. VANDE WIELE. 1972. Endocrinology **90:** 1133.
7. CSAPO, A. I., F. DRAY & T. ERDOS. 1975. Endocrinology **97:** 603.
8. WIEST, W. G. 1963. J. Biol. Chem. **238:** 94.
9. WIEST, W. G. 1963. Endocrinology **73:** 310.
10. ARMSTRONG, D. R. & E. R. KING. 1971. Endocrinology **89:** 191.
11. SAFFRAN, J., B. K. LOESER, B. M. HAAS & H. E. STAVELY. 1974. Steroids **34:** 839.
12. REDMOND, A. F. & G. J. PEPE. 1985. Biol. Reprod. **32:** (suppl. 1) 130. Abstract #185.
13. MALLONEE, R. C. & J. M. YOCHIM. 1979. J. Steroid Biochem. **11:** 745.
14. CUMMINGS, A. M. & J. M. YOCHIM. 1984. J. Theor. Biol. **106:** 353.
15. MULDOON, T. G. 1980. Endocrin. Rev. **1:** 339.
16. WALTERS, M. R. & J. H. CLARK. 1978. Endocrinology **103:** 601.
17. WALTERS, M. R. & J. H. CLARK. 1979. Endocrinology **105:** 382.
18. OKULICZ, W. C., R. W. EVANS & W. W. LEAVITT. 1981. Steroids **37:** 463.
19. LEAVITT, W. W. 1985. Endocrinology **116:** 1079.
20. MIURA, S., L. BURZIO & S. S. KOIDE. 1972. Horm. Metab. Res. **4:** 273.
21. MULLER, W. E. G., A. TOTSUKA, I. NUSER, J. OBERMEIEN, H. J. ROHDE & R. K. ZAHN. 1974. Nucleic Acids Res. **1:** 1317.
22. BRALEY, J. C., R. B. SANDERS & J. M. YOCHIM. Unpublished results.
23. CUMMINGS, A. M. & J. M. YOCHIM. 1983. Endocrinology **112:** 1412.
24. CUMMINGS, A. M. & J. M. YOCHIM. 1983. Endocrinology **112:** 1407.
25. MULLER, W. E. G., H. J. ROHDE & R. K. ZAHN. 1976. Biochimie **58:** 543.
26. OKA, H. & J. B. FIELD 1968. J. Biol. Chem. **243:** 815.
27. MANDEL, P., C. NIEDERGANG & H. OKAZAKI. 1980. Dev. Cell Biol. **6:** 21.
28. MALLONEE, R. C. & J. M. YOCHIM. 1980. Biol. Reprod. **23:** 588.
29. YOCHIM. J. M. & R. C. MALLONEE. 1980. Biol. Reprod. **23:** 595.
30. MARCUS, G. J. 1974. Biol. Reprod. **10:** 447.
31. GERSCHENSON, L. E., E. CONNER & J. T. MURAI. 1977. Endocrinology **100:** 1468.
32. YOCHIM. J. M. 1984. Biol. Reprod. **30:** 637.
33. YOCHIM. J. M. & V. J. DE FEO. 1963. Endocrinology **72:** 317.
34. ROTHCHILD, I. & R. K. MEYER. 1942. Physiol. Zool. **15:** 216.
35. SALDARINI, R. J. & J. M. YOCHIM. 1967. Endocrinology **80:** 453.
36. YOCHIM, J. M. & G. J. PEPE. 1971. Biol. Reprod. **5:** 172.
37. LEROY, F., J. VANSANDE, G. SHETGEN & D. BRESSEUR. 1974. J. Reprod. Fertil. **39:** 207.
38. RANKIN, J. C., B. E. LEDFORD & B. BAGGETT. 1977. Biol. Reprod. **17:** 549.
39. BEKAIRI, A. M., R. B. SANDERS & J. M. YOCHIM. 1984. Biol. Reprod. **31:** 742.
40. BEKAIRI, A. M., R. B. SANDERS, F. S. ABULABAN & J. M. YOCHIM. 1984. Biol. Reprod. **31:** 752.
41. SANDERS, R. B., A. M. BEKAIRI & J. M. YOCHIM. 1984. Fed. Proc. Fed. Am. Soc. Exp. Biol. **43:** 1583. Abstr. #971.
42. MOSS, J. & M. VAUGHAN. 1978. Proc. Nat. Acad. Sci. USA **75:** 3621.
43. AURBACH, G. D. 1982. Annu. Rev. Physiol. **44:** 653.
44. BLOMQUIST, C. H. 1973. J. Biol. Chem. **248:** 7044.

Progesterone Regulation of Protein Synthesis and Steroid Receptor Levels in Decidual Cells[a]

WENDELL W. LEAVITT, AKIHIRO TAKEDA, AND
RICHARD G. MacDONALD[b]

Department of Biochemistry
Texas Tech University Health Sciences Center
Lubbock, Texas 79430

INTRODUCTION

Steroid hormones influence gene transcription in target cells through a process involving hormone binding to specific intracellular receptor proteins.[1,2] Much has been learned about the macromolecular events regulated by steroid hormones in target cells that synthesize and secrete hormone-specific protein products, and progesterone action can be attributed to the regulation of gene expression and the formation of specific messenger RNA molecules for these export proteins.[3] The nature of the interaction between the receptor-hormone complex and the acceptor (effector) sites in the target cell nucleus that control gene expression, however, remains largely unknown. It is generally believed that a relationship must exist between the number of nuclear receptor sites and hormone-dependent gene transcription.[4] Evidence is needed to verify, however, that such a relationship actually exists, and it is not certain whether hormone action is the result of receptor binding and retention by nuclear acceptor sites,[3,4] receptor "processing" in the nucleus,[5,6] or other events.[7] Thus, we need to learn more about receptor regulation and processing in order to learn how hormone action is mediated at the level of gene expression.

In this chapter, we will review new approaches to the study of progesterone action in the decidualized rodent uterus. Implantation of the blastocyst in the wall of the sensitized uterus leads to proliferation of the underlying endometrial stromal cells to form the decidua. The decidual reaction can be induced experimentally to form "deciduoma" in the absence of a fertilized ovum by traumatization of the endometrium during the sensitive period. A unique feature of the deciduomal reaction in the rodent uterus is that pro-

[a] This work was supported by NIH Grants HD18711 and HD18712.

[b] Present address: Department of Biochemistry, University of Massachusetts Medical Center, Worcester, Massachusetts 01605.

gesterone is required for the initial stromal cell response and for maintenance of the proliferated state of the endometrium.[8,9] Thus, the artificially decidualized hamster uterus is an ideal model system for studying the biochemical changes and alterations in specific gene expression during proliferation and differentiation of a progesterone-dominated tissue independent of estrogen action.[8]

One hormone may act to alter the expression of another hormone, and the modulation of estrogen action by progesterone in target cells of the female reproductive tract is a classic example of this phenomenon. The underlying mechanism responsible for progesterone-induced changes in estrogen action, however, is unknown. It may be pertinent that progesterone down regulates the estrogen receptor (Re) system,[10] and the site of progesterone action appears to reside in the target cell nucleus.[11,12] Recently, we noted that progesterone mediates a selective loss of the occupied form of Re from the target cell nucleus,[13] and our studies with the estrogen-primed rodent uterus suggested that progesterone promotes nuclear Re turnover by a process involving a receptor regulatory factor that may function to release Re from nuclear acceptor sites and thereby modify estrogen-dependent gene expression.[14,15] This chapter will present new information on steroid receptor regulation in decidual cells. Because the progesterone receptor (Rp) response to progesterone withdrawal *in vivo* is compromised by the rapid regression of deciduomal tissue, decidual cell cultures were used to study Re and Rp recovery following progesterone withdrawal *in vitro*. The results show that progesterone down regulates both Re and Rp in hamster decidual cells. Recent studies on the receptors for several hormones[16–20] have demonstrated the utility of the density-shift technique for monitoring receptor protein dynamics. Thus, we have employed the density-shift method to determine whether progesterone controls Re turnover and/or synthesis in hamster decidual cells. We have recently developed conditions for growing hamster decidual cells in primary culture,[21] and these cells contain Re in addition to Rp when cultured in the absence of steroid hormones.[22] Using the density-shift method, we found that the down regulation of nuclear Re induced by progesterone is indeed the result of an acceleration in the turnover (processing) of preexisting receptor followed by an inhibition of E_2-induced receptor synthesis. We propose that this mechanism may account for the down regulation of uterine Re under physiological conditions such as pregnancy where progesterone action predominates over that of estrogen.

EXPERIMENTAL

Protein Synthesis in the Decidualized Uterus

Maintenance of the differentiated state of the endometrial stromal cells in the experimentally decidualized uterus requires progesterone action.[9]

Hence, it is not feasible to study the synthesis of progesterone-specific uterine proteins during pseudopregnancy in a direct manner, that is, following progesterone administration to progesterone-deficient animals. Our approach to this problem was to maintain the decidualized state of the uterus in ovariectomized, pseudopregnant hamsters through implantation of Silastic pellets containing progesterone. Then, progesterone-dependent changes in protein synthesis could be assessed after hormone withdrawal. The hormone implants were removed from one set of animals (progesterone withdrawn), and the synthesis of uterine proteins was measured 8 h later by labeling with [^{35}S]methionine in vitro followed by two-dimensional gel electrophoresis.[8] Pseudopregnant hamsters that retained the progesterone implants served as paired controls for the progesterone-withdrawn animals.

FIGURE 1 shows the effect of progesterone withdrawal on synthesis of proteins in deciduomal cytosol on day 7 of pseudopregnancy. The top panel shows proteins from control tissue, whereas the lower panel represents proteins from the progesterone-withdrawn uterus. Note that labeled acidic proteins are well distributed throughout the pH range 5.5 to 6.8. Many basic proteins that fail to migrate into the first-dimensional (IEF) gel are found along the right-hand edge of the second-dimensional (SDS-PAGE) gel. The most heavily labeled protein spot in all the gels is actin.[8] This autoradiographic spot corresponds to the major Coomassie blue-staining protein, and the intensity of the actin spot is not affected by progesterone withdrawal and serves as an indicator of the degree of film exposure in paired autoradiograms.

Progesterone withdrawal produced changes in intensity of at least 29 different protein spots in deciduomal cytosol. Of these 29 changes, 16 decreased in spot intensity, suggesting that progesterone is needed for enhanced synthesis of these proteins during pseudopregnancy. The other 13 spots showed increased intensity after 8 h of progesterone withdrawal, indicating that progesterone action also decreases or represses synthesis of certain proteins. The degree of spot-intensity changes varied as a function of progesterone withdrawal. At the extremes, withdrawal of progesterone produced virtual elimination of some spots (e.g., spots 3,5,8,16,19,20 in FIG. 1) and appearance of others (spots 21,27,28). A detailed list of molecular parameters and intensity changes for the progesterone-dependent proteins in deciduomal cytosol is reported elsewhere.[8]

An interesting feature of the autoradiograms shown in FIGURE 1 is the apparently coordinate repression by progesterone of the protein(s) represented by spots 23, 25, and 29. These spots form a "belt", representing a series of spots differing slightly in charge and molecular weight that behave similarly in response to hormonal stimulus. These characteristics have been described by Ivarie and O'Farrell[23] as resulting from discrete posttranslational modifications of a single protein, perhaps by glycosylation or some other mechanism.

Progesterone withdrawal also produced changes in synthesis of nuclear acidic proteins that were extracted from deciduomal nuclei with detergent (FIG. 1). As in the deciduomal cytosol, these intensity changes occurred in both directions. Increases in spot intensity dominated in the deciduomal

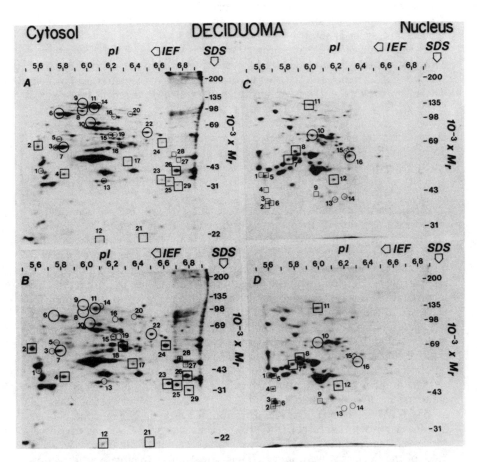

FIGURE 1. Effects of progesterone (P) withdrawal on synthesis of specific proteins in hamster deciduoma. Deciduomal tissues from control and P-withdrawn (8 h) hamsters were labeled with [^{35}S]methionine *in vitro*. Panels **A** and **B**: Cytosol proteins. Cytosol was prepared from control (**A**) and progesterone-withdrawn (**B**) hamsters and assayed for incorporation of label by precipitation with trichloroacetic acid. The cytosols applied to the first-dimensional isoelectric focusing gels each contained 5×10^4 cpm in volumes of 40 μl (**A**) and 90 μl (**B**). Two-dimensional gel electrophoresis and autoradiography were done as described elsewhere.[8] Film was exposed to the dried gels for 11 days. Panels **C** and **D**: Nuclear proteins. The nuclear extracts applied to the isoelectric focusing gels contained 5×10^4 cpm in 120 μl (control, **C**) and 196 μl (P-withdrawn, **D**). Film was exposed to the dried two-dimensional gels for 7 days. Squares enclose spots that increased in intensity after progesterone withdrawal; circles enclose spots that decrease in intensity after withdrawal.[8]

nucleus ($^{11}/_{16}$ increases, $^5/_{16}$ decreases) as compared to the cytosol, in which the direction of changes was more balanced ($^{13}/_{29}$ increase, $^{16}/_{29}$ decreases). The nuclear proteins extracted under these conditions are mostly acidic, and few, if any, basic proteins are found in the nuclear extract. The major, heavily labeled spot again is actin.

Fewer changes in specific protein synthesis occurred upon progesterone withdrawal on day 7 in myometrial cytosol compared to deciduomal cytosol.[8] Despite this difference and the obvious dissimilarities in the patterns of protein labeling in these two tissues, intensity changes also occurred in myometrial cytosol. Many of the heavily labeled proteins extracted from the myometrial nucleus were the same as those in the deciduomal nuclear extract, but few of these protein spots were affected by progesterone withdrawal. There was no overlap between the intensity changes observed in deciduomal and myometrial nuclei. In sharp contrast to the preponderance of increases in spot intensity in the deciduomal nucleus, decreases in spot intensity prevailed in the myometrial nucleus ($^9/_{11}$ decreases, $^2/_{11}$ increases).

Progesterone-dependent changes in specific protein synthesis were determined as a function of time during decidualization in both the deciduoma and myometrium.[8] In deciduomal cytosol, the number of progesterone-dependent changes in specific protein synthesis was smallest on day 6, increased on day 7, and then decreased somewhat on day 8. These variations in hormonal response were consistent with the progesterone-dependence of [^{35}S]methionine incorporation for the deciduomal cytosol. The majority of spot intensity increases in the deciduomal cytosol were minor, whereas intensity decreases were predominantly major in degree. The direction of response to progesterone withdrawal in this tissue shifted progressively with time, from a predominantly positive character (8 increases, 3 decreases) on day 6 toward a more negative one (8 increases, 12 decreases) on day 8.

The number of progesterone-dependent spot intensity changes in the deciduomal nucleus decreased with time of pseudopregnancy, being maximal on day 6 (27 total changes). The direction of synthetic changes for nuclear deciduomal proteins in response to progesterone withdrawal was very positive. Moreover, many of the spot intensity increases were major in degree, whereas most of the decreases were minor. Thus, the number, degree, and direction of progesterone withdrawal-induced changes in synthesis of deciduomal proteins varied depending on time during pseudopregnancy.

There were fewer hormone-dependent spot intensity changes among proteins from the myometrium than in the deciduoma.[8] Moreover, many of the characteristics of the response to progesterone withdrawal differed markedly in the two tissues. The response of proteins in myometrial cytosol was consistently negative over the course of the experiment, and the degree of these changes was mostly minor. Furthermore, few increases in specific protein synthesis were observed upon progesterone withdrawal in the myometrial nucleus. The number of spot intensity increases did not vary substantially on different days of pseudopregnancy. Decreases in spot intensity, however, did occur in the myometrial nucleus, some of which were major in degree.

Deciduomal Marker Proteins

Two-dimensional electrophoresis of nuclear extract containing 15 μg of protein and subsequent staining resolved more than 500 polypeptide spots.[21] Because our objective was to identify markers of decidualization, we required that a marker protein had to respond consistently in deciduoma as compared to nondecidualized endometrium. By necessity, this approach eliminated those proteins that responded in some but not all cases, and we found 11 deciduoma-associated proteins, the amount or staining intensity of which were different

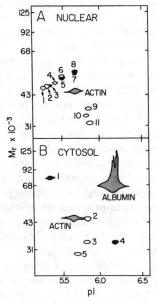

FIGURE 2. Schematic representation of nuclear (**A**) and cytosolic (**B**) deciduoma-associated proteins identified by two-dimensional gel electrophoresis. Spots represent deciduoma-associated proteins: solid symbols = deciduomal specific; open symbols = growth related (found in fetal fibroblast cultures).[21]

from that of the nondecidualized endometrial samples. A qualitative change was defined as the appearance of a spot that did not exist in the gel of the nondecidualized endometrium, and a quantitative change was defined as a twofold or greater increase in the size and intensity of a spot.

The nuclear deciduoma-associated proteins are illustrated in FIGURE 2. Two-dimensional gels from deciduoma and 48 h decidual cell cultures showed that most proteins could be arranged in two groups; within each group the proteins had similar pI, M_r, and color. Proteins 1-8 were light brown, and proteins 9-11 were black. The characteristics of these 11 proteins were consistent from gel to gel and from sample to sample both *in vivo* and in nuclear extracts of decidual cell cultures.

Those proteins that we have designated deciduoma-associated proteins were consistently observed to change in each pair of gels surveyed. Some protein spots varied in size or intensity in an inconsistent manner and were excluded from analysis. In addition, some polypeptides were observed to decrease in size or intensity during decidualization, and these too were excluded from analysis.

The most intensely stained protein in these samples was actin (pI 5.74, M_r 44,500). This protein served as a reference for estimating the reproducibility of protein load and two-dimensional migration pattern. When comparing duplicate runs of the same sample, the reproducibility of the protein pattern was found to be greater than 99% for the 500 proteins resolved, that is, the protein patterns were identical when superimposed.

Because decidualization is characterized by rapid cellular growth, we reasoned that certain of these proteins could be growth related and might be found in other rapidly growing cells. Therefore, a monolayer culture of fetal fibroblasts from hamster embryos taken on day 8 of gestation was prepared, and nuclear proteins were analyzed as described for decidual cultures. The three black proteins (spots 9-11), and four brown proteins (spots 1,2,4, and 5) were present in these rapidly proliferating fibroblast cultures (FIG. 2). Thus, seven of the deciduoma-associated proteins were also present in nondecidual cells undergoing rapid growth. Four nuclear proteins, however, were deciduoma specific, unrelated to growth of fetal hamster fibroblasts.

Two-dimensional electrophoresis of cytosolic preparations and subsequent Gelcode staining resulted in approximately 400 stained protein spots.[21] Five proteins characteristic of decidualization were present on day 6, 7, and 8 in the decidualized uterus and in 48 h cell cultures (FIG. 2). In contrast to the nuclear deciduomal proteins, each of these 5 cytosolic proteins stained a different color and was widely separated from the others in pI and M_r. The cytosolic proteins were more evenly distributed throughout the ampholine pH range in the isoelectric focusing (IEF) dimension than were the nuclear samples, which were concentrated in the lower pI range. Approximately 95% of the proteins extracted from nuclei had pI values $\leq$ 7.1, and hence were resolved in these gels. By comparison, a larger percentage of cytosolic proteins had pI values $\geq$ 7.1 and therefore were excluded from analysis.

Serum proteins were analyzed on two-dimensional gels to control for any quantitative changes resulting from load differences due to varying degrees of serum contamination. Based on relative staining intensity of the major serum proteins (*e.g.*, albumin, pI 6.2, M_r 69,000), serum proteins were estimated to contribute approximately 25-33% of the total protein load in gels containing deciduomal cytosolic proteins (FIG. 2). This contamination was absent in cell cultures. All five deciduoma-associated proteins as defined *in vivo* are evident in cell culture cytosolic samples. Cytosolic protein samples from cultured fetal hamster fibroblasts were prepared, and three of the cytosolic proteins characteristic of the deciduoma were also detected in fibroblast cytosol. Thus, three of the deciduomal proteins appeared to be associated with the growth of fetal hamster fibroblasts, and two were deciduoma specific.

Receptor Regulation in Decidual Cells

Total Re and Rp were measured in the cytosol and nuclear fractions of hamster deciduomal tissue and decidual cell cultures. Correlation of serum steroid (estradiol and progesterone) and deciduomal receptor profiles revealed a significant loss of Re during the first four days of decidualization that was not attributable to changes in serum steroid levels. Ovarian hormone secretion during decidualization produced estradiol levels of 60-70 pg/ml serum and progesterone levels of 6-10 ng/ml serum from day 5 to day 8 (FIG. 3). On day 9, serum estradiol rose and progesterone fell, and extensive regressive changes occurred in the deciduoma. Although serum steroid titers remained fairly constant until day 8, deciduomal receptor levels changed significantly (p < 0.05) during this period (FIG. 4). Cytosol Re rose to a peak on day 6 and then decreased progressively from day 7 to day 9. Nuclear Re decreased successively on day 7, day 8, and reached nondetectable levels (< 50 fmol/

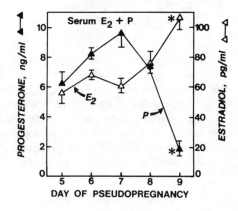

FIGURE 3. Serum estradiol (E$_2$) and progesterone (P) levels during decidualization in the pseudopregnant hamster. Serum steroids were determined by specific radioimmunoassay. Each point is the mean ± SEM (n = 10). *p < 0.05, Student-Newman-Keul's test.

mg DNA) on day 9. By contrast, Rp levels increased progressively from day 5 to day 8 in deciduomal cytosol and nucleus, and then Rp fell precipitously in both cellular fractions on day 9 (FIG. 4) in association with deciduomal regression.

To determine the response of the deciduomal Rp system to the withdrawal of ovarian steroid hormones, animals were ovariectomized (ovex) at 1000 h on day 6, and cytosol and nuclear Rp levels were measured at 4 h, 8 h, 16 h, and 24 h after ovex. Control animals were subjected to a sham ovex procedure and studied at the same intervals. At 4 h after ovex, nuclear Rp decreased, and cytosol Rp did not change as compared to the sham control (FIG. 5). Nuclear Rp remained low from 4 h to 24 hours. Cytosol Rp increased twofold, however, from 4 h to 8 h before declining progressively at 16 h and 24 h after ovex. The accumulation of cytosol Rp beyond 8 h appeared to be compromised by deciduomal involution that occurred at 16 h and 24 h after ovex.

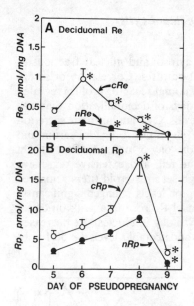

FIGURE 4. Estrogen receptor (Re) and progesterone receptor (Rp) levels in cytosol (c) and nuclear (n) fractions of the hamster deciduoma. Each point is the mean ± SEM (n = 10). *p < 0.05, Student-Newman-Keul's test.

A decidual-cell tissue culture system was used to study the receptor recovery response to progesterone withdrawal. Decidual cell cultures were initiated at 20 h after deciduomal induction, and most decidual cells adhered to the culture dish within 2 h after seeding. After 48 h of culture, monolayers of large polymorphic decidual cells were obtained, and most cells were binucleate with two or more nucleoli per nucleus (FIG. 6).

We studied the effect of progesterone on the growth of decidual cell cultures and discovered that progesterone was not required for decidual cell

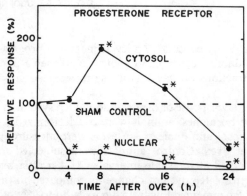

FIGURE 5. Deciduomal progesterone receptor (Rp) response to ovariectomy (ovex) on day 6 of pseudopregnancy. The Rp response of ovex animals is plotted relative to Rp values for sham-operated controls. *p < 0.05 versus sham control. Deciduomal regression commenced between 8 h and 16 h after ovex.

proliferation (FIG. 7). In fact, decidual cell numbers appeared to be somewhat lower in cultures grown with progesterone than without it (FIG. 7). Examination of these cultures by phase contrast microscopy revealed no discernible change in decidual cell morphology that could be attributed to progesterone withdrawal.

Because decidual cells could be maintained in tissue culture in the absence of progesterone, it was possible to study Rp and Re responses to progesterone

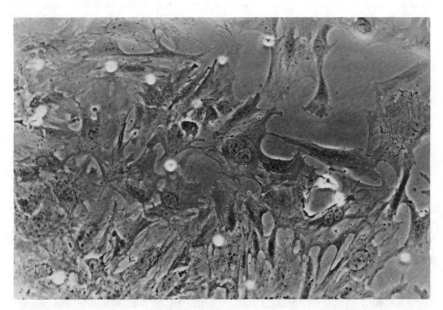

FIGURE 6. Phase contrast microscopy of decidual cells at 48 h of culture. The procedure used for the isolation and culture of hamster decidual cells is as described by Leavitt *et al.*[21] At 18 h after deciduomal induction, the endometrium was removed, and cells were obtained after 2 h of collagenase digestion. Cells were dispersed, pelleted by centrifugation, and resuspended in complete medium (Ham's F-12/Dulbecco's modified Eagle's medium (1:1) containing 5% dextran-coated charcoal-stripped horse serum, 100 U penicillin/ml, 100 μg streptomycin/ml, 5 μg insulin/ml, 5 μg transferrin/ml, 5 ng selenium/ml, and 10 ng progesterone/ml). Cells were plated at 5 × 10^5 cells/dish and incubated in a humidified atmosphere of 95% air/5% CO_2 at 37° C. Erythrocytes and unattached cells were removed by changing the medium at 2 h after plating leaving a homogeneous population of decidual cells attached to the dish. The medium was changed every 24 h thereafter. Microscopy taken with a Nikon Diaphot-TMD inverted microscope (x 280).

withdrawal *in vitro*. At 72 h of culture in medium containing progesterone, only Rp was detectable in decidual cells (FIG. 8). Re was not detectable (<200 fmol/mg DNA) in either cytosol or nuclei from cells grown with progesterone. When progesterone was removed from the medium, however, cytosol Re recovered with time of culture from 8 h to 16 h (FIG. 8). Progesterone withdrawal also caused parallel increases in cytosol and nuclear

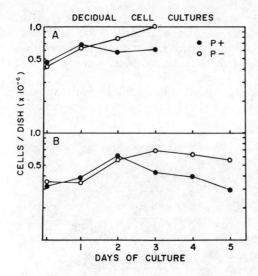

FIGURE 7. Growth of decidual cell cultures with and without progesterone (P, 10 ng/ml). Cultures were seeded with 5×10^5 cells/dish at time 0. The first point represents the number of decidual cells that had attached at 2 hours. Cells were dispersed using 0.5% trypsin and counted with a hemacytometer. Each point is the mean of three dishes.

Rp, and estradiol treatment (8 nM) in combination with progesterone withdrawal further enhanced Rp levels in decidual cell cultures. These results with cultured decidual cells demonstrate that (1) progesterone down regulates Re and Rp, (2) Re recovers rapidly upon progesterone withdrawal, and (3) the Re system is competent to respond to estrogen action in terms of Rp induction. Thus, decidual cell cultures can serve as a model system to study the up and down regulation of Re and Rp systems.

In our previous work, the amount of receptor present at a given time was measured with binding assays that did not permit estimation of receptor turnover and synthesis rates. Thus, in order to further evaluate the re-regulatory factor (ReRF) hypothesis, a method was needed that would directly assess receptor protein dynamics. Recent studies on the receptors for thyroid hormone, glucocorticoid and estrogen, have demonstrated the utility of the density-shift method for measuring receptor turnover.[16–20] Therefore, we decided to use this method to determine whether progesterone controls Re turnover and/or synthesis in hamster decidual cells.

With the density-shift method, cells are first incubated in medium containing normal [^{1}H ^{12}C ^{14}N]amino acids, and then they are switched to medium supplemented with dense [^{2}H ^{13}C ^{15}N]amino acids. After various periods of incubation, the nascent proteins synthesized from dense amino acids are separated from the preexisting proteins of normal density by sucrose density-gradient centrifugation. The newly synthesized Re sediments faster into the gradient than does preexisting Re, and measurement of the two resultant receptor peaks permits estimation of Re synthesis and degradation, respectively.[20]

Primary cultures of hamster decidual cells were grown for two days in medium containing normal amino acids.[21] Then at time 0, the cultures were switched to medium supplemented with dense amino acids and incubated with either 1 nM estradiol (E_2) or 1 nM estradiol plus 100 nM progesterone (E_2 + P). Cells were harvested at 1, 3, 6, and 9 h of incubation with steroid hormone and dense amino acids, and nuclear Re was extracted with 10 mM pyridoxal phosphate and labeled with [^{125}I]estradiol. Labeled receptor peaks were resolved by centrifugation at 0° C for 38 h in 5-20% sucrose gradients.

The receptor peak of normal density decreased with time of incubation (FIG. 9), and the half-life ($t\frac{1}{2}$) of preexisting receptor was estimated from the disappearance rate of the normal-density receptor peak (FIG. 10). For E_2-treated decidual cells, the $t\frac{1}{2}$ of nuclear Re was 3.7 h, which is in agreement with $t\frac{1}{2}$ values (3.0-4.0 h) reported for Re in MCF-7 breast cancer cells using this same method.[20] By contrast, E_2 + P treatment caused nuclear Re of normal density to turn over twice as rapidly as compared to E_2 alone. There was a significant (p < 0.05) enhancement of Re turnover at 3, 6, and 9 h of E_2 + P treatment, with an attendant decrease in Re half-life from 3.7 h (E_2) to 1.9 h (E_2 + P) (FIG. 10).

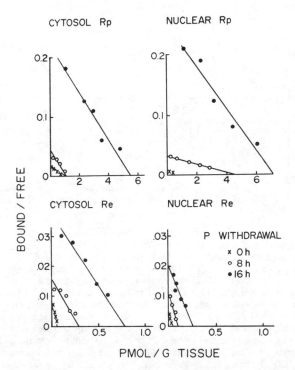

FIGURE 8. Scatchard plots of specific binding data for progesterone receptor (Rp) and estrogen receptor (Re) assays done on cytosol and nuclear fractions derived from decidual cells at 0 h, 8 h, and 16 h following progesterone (P) withdrawal. Decidual cells were harvested at 72 h of culture. Progesterone withdrawal was accomplished by changing the medium at 8 h or 16 h before harvesting. The Scatchard plots show a progressive increase in Rp and Re concentration with time of P withdrawal.

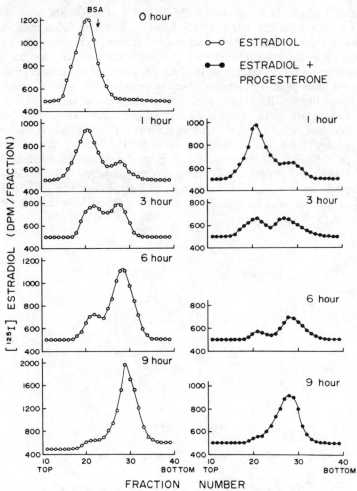

FIGURE 9. Separation of normal and dense nuclear estrogen receptors (Re) by sucrose density-gradient centrifugation after incubation of hamster decidual cells with dense amino acids and either 1 nM 17β-estradiol (E_2) or 1 nM E_2 plus 100 nM progesterone (P). Decidual cell cultures were grown for two days, the medium was replaced with normal amino acid medium containing 1 nM E_2, and cells were incubated for 1 hour. This E_2 pretreatment was done to charge unfilled Re sites. At time 0, normal medium was replaced with dense amino acid medium containing either 1 nM E_2 or 1 nM E_2 plus 100 nM P. The cells were cultured for 1, 3, 6, and 9 h before harvesting. At the indicated times, dense amino acid medium was decanted, and cells were washed twice with ice-cold buffered saline. The cells were removed from the dish, collected by low speed centrifugation and homogenized in barbital buffer (20 mM sodium barbital, 5 mM dithiothreitol, 10% glycerol, pH 8.0). After centrifugation at 800 × g for 10 min, the nuclear pellet was washed twice with barbital buffer, and nuclear Re was extracted with 10 mM pyridoxal 5'-phosphate in barbital buffer for 1 hour. The nuclear Re was labeled with 5 nM [^{125}I]16α-iodoestradiol (2200 Ci/mmol) and, after removing free steroid by treatment with dextran-coated charcoal, an aliquot was layered on the top of a 5-20% sucrose gradient and centrifuged at 357,000 × g for 33 hours. Two-drop fractions were collected and counted at 76% efficiency. The gradient profile was corrected for nonspecific binding (competed sample) providing the specific [^{125}I]iodoestradiol binding data plotted here. Bovine serum albumin (BSA) was used as a sedimentation marker (4.6S).

The newly synthesized Re, which incorporated dense amino acids, was apparent within 1 h of incubation as a second, faster-sedimenting peak that accumulated with time of incubation up to 9 h (FIG. 9). The size of the newly synthesized Re peak was smaller in the E_2 + P treatment as compared to E_2 at 3, 6, and 9 h (FIG. 9), but this does not necessarily represent a decrease in synthesis because Re turnover had increased. In fact, when Re synthesis

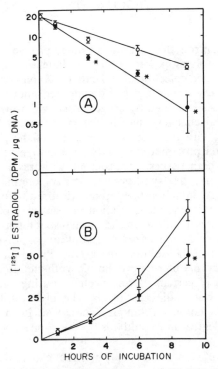

FIGURE 10. Turnover of estrogen receptor (Re) of normal density (panel **A**) and synthesis of dense Re (panel **B**) in decidual cells cultured with dense amino acids and either 1 nM estradiol (E_2) (○) or 1 nM E_2 plus 100 nM progesterone (P) (●). Normal and dense Re were separated and quantitated as shown in FIGURE 9. **A.** The log of the normal-density Re peak (dpm/μg DNA, mean ± SEM) was plotted versus time, and the regression line was calculated by the least squares method. The half-life ($t\frac{1}{2}$) of preexisting Re was extrapolated from the regression lines: E_2 = 3.7 h (r = 0.92, n = 16); E_2 + P = 1.9 h (r = 0.95, n = 14). **B.** The synthesis of dense amino acid-labeled Re (dpm/μg DNA, mean ± SEM) was calculated with the formula (K_s · t) where K_s = the rate of synthesis (dpm/μg DNA · hour) and t = time (hours). *Significantly different (p < 0.05), E_2 versus E_2 + P, Student's *t* test.

was corrected for the change in turnover by the method of Schimke[24] (FIG. 10), the rate of Re synthesis was unchanged in E_2 + P cells, and in E_2 cells it increased from 4.6 ± 0.4 (mean ± SEM) at 1 h to 8.5 ± 0.7 dpm/μg DNA · hour at 9 h of incubation. Thus, although progesterone did not significantly alter the basal rate of Re synthesis, it did block E_2-induced stimulation of Re synthesis at 9 h (FIG. 10).

This experiment demonstrates unequivocally that the down regulation of nuclear estrogen receptor induced by progesterone is indeed the result of an acceleration in the turnover (processing) of preexisting Re followed by an inhibition of E_2-induced receptor synthesis.

DISCUSSION

Progesterone controls the synthesis of many proteins in the decidualized uterus. The high resolving power of the two-dimensional gel electrophoresis technique has permitted detection of 500 individual components in deciduomal and myometrial cytosols. On day 7 of pseudopregnancy, the number of proteins whose synthesis is altered by progesterone withdrawal is greater in the deciduoma (45 total changes) than in the myometrium (26 changes). This result is consistent with the greater dependence of the proliferated state of the endometrium on progesterone relative to the myometrium during pseudopregnancy.[28] In both tissues, progesterone withdrawal predominantly induced decreases in the synthesis of many uterine proteins during pseudopregnancy. Although progesterone withdrawal for 8 h produced a decrease in [35S]methionine incorporation on each day of pseudopregnancy studied, both increases and decreases in protein spot intensity were observed.[8] This observation further emphasizes the complexity of progesterone regulation of protein synthesis in the decidualized uterus. Progesterone is required for maintenance of maximal uterine protein biosynthetic rates, yet the hormone represses synthesis of certain uterine proteins during decidualization. This important finding was made possible by the high resolution of the two-dimensional electrophoretic technique. These spot intensity increases were mostly minor in degree and could easily have gone undetected in one-dimensional gels.

The "domain" of response to an effector that evokes many changes within a cell has been defined as the set of protein synthetic events that occur in response to the effector.[29] Ivarie and O'Farrell[23] described the glucocorticoid domains in two hepatoma cell lines using two-dimensional gel electrophoresis to identify the protein synthetic events that constitute those domains. According to O'Farrell and Ivarie,[30] a domain has the following properties: size, or the total number of events in the domain; heterogeneity, that is, direction of response for a given event; and overlap, or those events that, as a subset of a particular domain, are common to other domain(s). Within the limits of resolution of the present methodology, we have described the progesterone domains of response in the decidualized hamster uterus on days 6, 7, and 8 of pseudopregnancy. In both the deciduoma and myometrium, the domains of response change from day to day in both size and degree of overlap (FIG. 11), that is, whether the synthesis of a particular protein is under progesterone control, and to what extent, depends strongly on time during pseudopregnancy. These variations are illustrated schematically in FIGURE 11.

The overlapping regions of the rectangles (daily domains) in these diagrams represent the number of polypeptides whose synthesis was altered by progesterone withdrawal on more than one day of pseudopregnancy. Nonoverlapping areas indicate those protein synthetic changes that occurred exclusively on each day. Comparing the two tissues, overlap of the domains on successive days was remarkably similar among cytosolic proteins but drastically different in the nucleus. The overlapping subsets of the cytosolic domains were similar in size in the deciduoma and myometrium, but the individual polypeptides in these subsets were not the same. Thus, the shifts in the progesterone domains in the cytosol of both uterine tissues were not

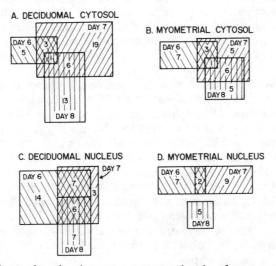

FIGURE 11. Temporal overlaps between progesterone domains of response on days 6, 7, and 8 of pseudopregnancy. Domains are represented by squares or rectangles whose area is proportional to the size of the domain, that is, the total of autoradiographic spot intensity changes produced by progesterone withdrawal on that day. Cross-hatched regions show the extent of overlap, representing proteins common to the domains on different days. The numbers within each region indicate the number of spots in each subset of the domains.[8] The term domain refers to those protein synthetic events occurring in response to the effector, progesterone, in accordance with its original usage in a similar context by Tomkins[29] and by Ivarie and O'Farrell.[30]

abrupt, but occurred gradually with some intensity changes occurring repeatedly over the three-day period of study. One protein spot in each tissue changed on all three days of the experiment, and these two proteins were dissimilar in terms of their pI/M_r values and direction of response.

Overlap of the daily domains in the deciduomal nucleus was extensive (FIG. 11). Nearly every protein spot that was affected by progesterone withdrawal on day 7 also was altered on day 6 or day 8 or both. Six protein spots changed on every day of the experiment in the deciduomal nucleus. These proteins differed substantially in pI and M_r, and their further characterization would be of interest. The smallest overlap between domains of response occurred in the myometrial nucleus. Minimal overlap was found on days 6 and 7, whereas the domain of response of day 8 was completely distinct from those of the previous two days. Finally, five proteins were found to overlap in the domains of response to progesterone withdrawal in deciduoma and myometrium. These findings suggest that, despite the substantial differences between the progesterone domains in these two tissues, there are some events common to both.

Progesterone-dependent alterations in synthesis of uterine proteins during decidualization reflect complex hormonal regulation of uterine gene expression. Some caution, however, should be exercised because the sensitivity of the two-dimensional gel electrophoretic system is such that small modifications in a protein can result in displacement of the protein from one location on the gel to another. Thus, progesterone-induced alterations in the activity or specificity of enzymes involved in posttranslational modification of proteins could be responsible for some of the effects we have observed on specific protein labeling in the decidualized uterus. A progesterone-dependent change in the degradative rate of a specific protein might be manifested as a decreased intensity in that spot coupled with the possible appearance of two or more spots having different pI values and lower M_r than the parent protein. Examination of the autoradiographic maps for cytosolic proteins (FIG. 1) revealed that many of the spot intensity decreases due to progesterone withdrawal were in the high molecular weight region ($M_r \geq 50,000$), whereas many increases in spot intensity occurred at the bottom end of the M_r range. Thus, if progesterone suppresses degradation of uterine proteins, then one might expect that progesterone withdrawal would enhance proteolysis by removing the hormonal inhibition. Progesterone withdrawal during pseudopregnancy does lead to regression and, ultimately, involution of the deciduoma.[9] Further studies are needed to determine whether progesterone-dependent changes in proteolysis are responsible for some of the changes we have observed in the gel maps.

In summary, the decidualized hamster uterus is a useful model system for studying hormonal effects on gene expression in a rapidly differentiating tissue. Our studies suggest that progesterone action in the decidualized uterus differs somewhat from that in the chick oviduct. In the latter model system, progesterone effects on specific gene expression are largely dependent on estrogen-induced cytodifferention and growth of the oviduct.[1] By contrast, growth and differentiation of the decidualized hamster uterus depend primarily on progesterone, which controls this process through bidirectional changes in uterine gene expression. Alterations occur in the protein composition of deciduomal tissue during differentiation, and these proteins can serve as markers of decidualization and be used to study decidual cells under conditions of cell culture. Previous attempts to study decidualization in vitro were limited to morphological and ultrastructural descriptions.[31,32] We have identified 11 nuclear and 5 cytosolic deciduomal proteins that can serve as specific indicators of the differentiated state of the decidual cell.

The high resolution of two-dimensional gel electrophoresis combined with the ultrasensitive Gelcode staining method have allowed us to expand previous estimates of the number of proteins associated with the decidualization response in the rodent uterus.[33,34] In contrast to previous studies, the present approach has permitted estimation of the molecular weight and isoelectric point of each protein, an important first step toward further characterization and, ultimately, identification of these proteins. The added dimension of individual spot coloration provided by the Gelcode staining method greatly facilitates the distinction between proteins in a complex two-dimensional map from a crude extract. Color is especially useful in discriminating between serum contaminants and cellular proteins in gels of cytosol samples.

It is not clear whether any of the deciduoma-related proteins described previously[33,34] are the same as those we have identified. The two-dimensional protein maps reported for rat deciduomal tissue,[35] however, have a striking similarity to the gel patterns we obtained with the hamster deciduoma. We have divided the deciduoma-associated proteins into two populations, those associated with rapidly growing fetal fibroblasts and those associated with differentiation, the acquisition of biochemical and morphological features necessary to perform a specialized function. The fully differentiated decidual cell is large, polyploid, and multinucleate. Although the function of decidual cells is not known, they play an important role during placentation. Cell size and shape may be important to deciduomal cell function, and the occurrence of polyploidy and multinucleation is the result of DNA replication without subsequent cytokinesis. We provided evidence that some deciduoma-associated proteins are growth related, whereas others are not. These latter deciduoma-specific proteins may be involved in regulating decidual cell size and ploidy. It is possible that deciduoma-specific proteins could be responsible for inhibition of cytokinesis, for example, these proteins could inhibit assembly of cortical microfilaments or block the association of functional elements in the contractile ring. If the mitotic phase of the cell cycle is disrupted, and the cell advances to G_1, individual cell growth is maintained without an increase in cell number. Therefore, the deciduoma-associated proteins could be regulatory in nature and responsible for the acquisition of morphological characteristics attributed to the decidualized state.

The set of deciduoma-associated proteins described here (FIG. 2) will permit decidualization to be studied in molecular terms. The preparation of specific immunological probes to these proteins will allow the detailed study of deciduomal protein synthesis and other hormonally directed biochemical processes during decidualization of endometrial stromal cells in tissue culture. Progesterone appears to have a constitutive effect on the synthesis and accumulation of many deciduomal proteins, and this may represent an important mechanism for hormonal control of deciduomal growth and differentiation. Thus, it will be of interest to determine how progesterone influences the synthesis and turnover of specific gene products in decidual cells.

We found that decidual cells can serve as a useful paradigm for studying how progesterone controls the Re system. Other workers have shown that steroid hormones influence the turnover of their own receptors. Glucocorticoids[36] and estrogens[20] both enhance the turnover rate of their respective receptors, whereas androgens have the opposite effect.[37] This is the first report, however, to show that one steroid hormone, progesterone, can affect the dynamics of the receptor for another hormone, estrogen.

Using the density-shift method to measure Re turnover and synthesis in uterine decidual cells, we were able to reveal important features of the molecular mechanism responsible for progestin-induced down regulation of nuclear Re. Progesterone markedly stimulated the turnover of preexisting nuclear Re within 3 h, and the synthesis of new Re from dense amino acids was inhibited subsequent to the change in Re turnover. Thus, these results demonstrate for the first time a rapid primary effect of progestin on nuclear Re processing followed by a secondary inhibition of E_2-induced Re replenishment. We suggest that this mechanism may be responsible for the down regulation of uterine Re under physiological conditions such as pregnancy

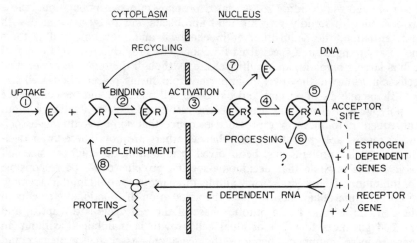

FIGURE 12. Estrogen receptor dynamics in the decidual cell. Steps are (1) hormone uptake by the cell, (2) binding to unoccupied receptor, (3) receptor activation, (4) binding to acceptor site, (5) receptor retention, (6) receptor processing, (7) receptor recycling, and (8) receptor replenishment. Abbreviations are E = estradiol-17β; R = estrogen receptor; A = nuclear acceptor site. Progesterone appears to act on steps 5 or 6.

were progesterone action predominates over that of estrogen. Progesterone not only suppresses Re but also inhibits other E_2-induced uterine proteins including the oxytocin receptor until the time of parturition.[25,26] Nuclear Re and E_2-dependent proteins, however can recover rapidly upon progesterone withdrawal,[26,27] showing that the inhibitory action of progesterone on nuclear Re retention is readily reversible. Thus, the stimulation of nuclear Re turnover may represent a fundamental mechanism responsible for progesterone modulation of E_2 action.

Our studies with the estrogen-primed rodent uterus suggested that progesterone promotes nuclear Re turnover by a process involving a progestin-induced factor (ReRF) that may function to release Re from nuclear acceptor sites and thereby modify estrogen-dependent gene expression (FIG. 12). Therefore, the progesterone-induced enhancement of nuclear Re turnover may be mediated by ReRF that is proposed to stimulate nuclear Re processing.[2] Although the mechanism of ReRF action is not known, previous studies with phosphatase inhibitors suggested that ReRF may be a nuclear phosphatase.[14,38] If true, progesterone may control Re retention by a dephosphorylation mechanism perhaps by ReRF action on either the Re protein or nuclear acceptor sites (or both), resulting in a destabilization of the Re molecule. Further work is in progress to elucidate the site and mechanism of ReRF action.

Decidualization of the rodent uterus is a classic response to progesterone action,[39] and in the hamster, decidual cell growth and differentiation are absolutely dependent upon progesterone.[28] Multiple progesterone-dependent changes occur in the synthesis of nuclear and cytosolic proteins in the hamster deciduoma,[8] and there is evidence for specific alterations in endometrial protein composition during deciduomal morphogenesis.[21] Presumably, hormone action is mediated by a specific Rp system present in hamster decidual tissue,[40] and the Re system is down regulated during decidualization (FIG. 4). Because Re levels decline to a greater extent in the deciduoma as compared to the myometrium,[9] it appears that the Re down regulation mechanism may be more effective in decidual cells than myometrial cells. Kimmel *et al.*[41] first noted in the rat that Re activity was less in deciduoma than in myometrium, and subsequent studies have confirmed that the number of Re sites diminishes during deciduomal development in the rat.[42-44] The loss of Re and retention of Rp sites appears to be a general phenomenon associated with decidual cell development in the rodent uterus, and this shift in the cellular receptor content may be related to the dominant role of progesterone in the decidualization process. Although it is tempting to suggest that receptor site availability may be important for the control of decidual cell responsiveness to hormone action, further studies are needed to establish that changes in receptor content actually do regulate the sensitivity of decidual cells to steroid hormone action.

REFERENCES

1. GRODY, W. W., W. T. SCHRADER & B. W. O'MALLEY. 1982. Activation, transformation and subunit structure of steroid hormone receptors. Endocrin. Rev. 3: 141-163.
2. LEAVITT, W. W., R. G. MACDONALD & W. C. OKULICZ. 1983. Hormonal regulation of estrogen and progesterone receptor systems. *In* Biochemical Action of Hormones. G. Litwack, Ed. Vol. 10: 324-356. Academic Press. New York.
3. SPELSBERG, T. C., B. A. LITTLEFIELD, R. SEELKE, G. N. DANI, H. TOYODA, P. BOYD-LEINEN, C. THRALL & O. L. KON. 1983. Role of specific chromosomal proteins and DNA sequences in the nuclear binding sites for steroid receptors. Recent Prog. Horm. Res. 39: 463-513.
4. JENSEN, E. V. 1979. Interaction of steroid hormones with the nucleus. Pharmacol. Rev. 30: 477-491.
5. HORWITZ, K. B. & W. L. MCGUIRE. 1978. Actinomyocin D prevents nuclear processing of estrogen receptor. J. Biol. Chem. 253: 6319-6322.
6. HORWITZ, K. B. & W. L. MCGUIRE. 1978. Nuclear mechanisms of estrogen action: Effects of estradiol and anti-estrogens on estrogen receptors in nuclear processing. J. Biol. Chem. 253: 8185-8191.

7. GORSKI, J., W. WELSHONS & D. SAKAI. 1984. Remodeling the estrogen receptor model. Mol. Cell. Endocrinol. 36: 11-15.
8. MACDONALD, R. G., K. O. MORENCY & W. W. LEAVITT. 1983. Progesterone modulation of specific protein synthesis in the decidualized hamster uterus. Biol. Reprod. 28: 753-766.
9. LEAVITT, W. W., T. J. CHEN & R. W. EVANS. 1979. Regulation and function of estrogen and progesterone receptor systems. In Steroid Hormone Receptor Systems. W. W. Leavitt & J. H. Clark, Eds.: 197-222. Plenum Press. New York.
10. CLARK, J. H., A. J. W. HSEUH & E. J. PECK JR. 1977. Regulation of estrogen receptor replenishment by progesterone. Ann. N.Y. Acad. Sci. 286: 161-178.
11. EVANS, R. W. & W. W. LEAVITT. 1980. Progesterone action in hamster uterus: rapid inhibition of ^{3}H-estradiol retention by the nuclear fraction. Endocrinology 107: 1261-1263.
12. EVANS, R. W. & W. W. LEAVITT. 1980. Progesterone inhibition of uterine nuclear estrogen receptor: dependence on RNA and protein synthesis. Proc. Natl. Acad. Sci. USA 77: 5856-5860.
13. OKULICZ, W. C., R. W. EVANS & W. W. LEAVITT. 1981. Progesterone regulation of the occupied form of nuclear estrogen receptor. Science 213: 1503-1505.
14. OKULICZ, W. C., R. G. MACDONALD & W. W. LEAVITT. 1981. Progesterone-induced estrogen receptor-regulatory factor in hamster uterine nuclei: preliminary characterization in a cell-free system. Endocrinology 109: 2273-2275.
15. MACDONALD, R. G., S. P. ROSENBERG & W. W. LEAVITT. 1983. Localization of estrogen receptor regulatory factor in the uterine nucleus. Mol. Cell. Endocrinol. 32: 301-313.
16. GARDNER, J. M. & D. M. FAMBROUGH. 1979. Acetylcholine receptor degradation measured by density labeling: effects of cholinergic ligands and evidence against recycling. Cell 16: 661-674.
17. REED, B. C. & M. D. LANE. 1980. Insulin receptor synthesis and turnover in differentiating 3T3-L1 preadipocytes. Proc. Natl. Acad. Sci. USA 77: 285-289.
18. RAAKA, B. M. & H. H. SAMUELS. 1981. Regulation of thyroid hormone nuclear receptor levels in GH1 cells by 3,5,3'-triiodo-L-thyronine. J. Biol. Chem. 256: 6883-6889.
19. RAAKA, B. M. & H. H. SAMUELS. 1983. The glucocorticoid receptor in GH1 cells. J. Biol. Chem. 258: 417-425.
20. ECKERT, R. L., A. MULLICK, E. A. RORKE & B. S. KATZENELLENBOGEN. 1984. Estrogen receptor synthesis and turnover in MCF-7 breast cancer cells measured by a density shift technique. Endocrinology 114: 629-637.
21. LEAVITT, W. W., R. G. MACDONALD & G. T. SHWAERY. 1985. Characterization of deciduoma marker proteins in hamster uterus: detection in decidual cell cultures. Biol. Reprod. 32: 631-643.
22. LEAVITT, W. W. 1984. Estrogen and progesterone receptors in decidual cells maintained in tissue culture. Biol. Reprod. 30(suppl. 1): 160.
23. IVARIE, R. D. & R. H. O'FARRELL. 1978. The glucocorticoid domain: steroid-mediated changes in the rate of synthesis of rat hepatoma proteins. Cell 13: 41-55.
24. SCHIMKE, R. T. 1975. Methods for analysis of enzyme synthesis and degradation in animal tissues. In Methods in Enzymology. B. W. O'Malley & J. G. HARDMAN, Eds. Vol. XL:241-266. Academic Press. New York.
25. ALEXANDROVA, M. & M. S. SOLOFF. 1980. Oxytocin receptors and parturition. I. Control of oxytocin receptor concentrations in the rat myometrium at term. Endocrinology 106: 730-735.
26. LEAVITT, W. W. 1985. Hormonal regulation of myometrial estrogen, progesterone, and oxytocin receptors in the pregnant and pseudopregnant hamster. Endocrinology 116: 1079-1084.
27. LEAVITT, W. W., W. C. OKULICZ, J. A. MCCRACKEN, W. SCHRAMM & W. F. ROBIDOUX JR. 1985. Rapid recovery of nuclear estrogen receptor and oxytocin receptor in the ovine uterus following progesterone withdrawal. J. Steroid Biochem. 22: 687-691.
28. BLAHA, G. C. & W. W. LEAVITT. 1978. Deciduomal responses in the uteri of ovariectomized golden hamster, comparing progesterone and three closely related steroids applied in utero. Biol. Reprod. 18: 441-447.
29. TOMKINS, G. M. 1975. The metabolic code: Biological symbolism and the origin of intracellular communication is discussed. Science 189: 760-763.

30. O'FARRELL, P. H. & R. D. IVARIE. 1979. The glucocorticoid domain of response: Measurement of pleiotropic cellular responses by two-dimensional gel electrophoresis. *In* Glucocorticoid Hormone Action. J. D. Baxter & G. G. Rousseau, Eds.: 189-201. Springer-Verlag. New York.

31. VLADIMIRSKY, F., L. CHEN, A. AMSTERDAM, U. ZOR & H. R. LINDER. 1977. Differentiation of decidual cells in cultures of rat endometrium. J. Reprod. Fertil. **49:** 61-68.

32. SANANES, N., S. WEILLER, E. BAULIEU & C. LEGOASCOGNE. 1978. *In vitro* decidualization of rat endometrial cells. Endocrinology **104:** 86-95.

33. DENARI, J. H. & J. M. ROSNER. 1978. Studies on biochemical characteristics of an early decidual protein. Int. J. Fertil. **23:** 123-127.

34. BELL, S. C. 1979. Synthesis of 'decidualization-associated proteins' in tissues of the rat uterus and placenta during pregnancy. J. Reprod. Fertil. **56:** 255-262.

35. LEJEUNE, B., R. LECOCQ, F. LAMY & F. LEROY. 1982. Changes in the pattern of endometrial protein synthesis during decidualization in the rat. J. Reprod. Fertil. **66:** 519-523.

36. MCINTYRE, W. R. & H. H. SAMUELS. 1985. Triamcinolone acetonide regulates glucocorticoid-receptor levels by decreasing the half-life of the activated nuclear-receptor form. J. Biol. Chem. **260:** 418-427.

37. SYMS, A. J., J. S. NORRIS, W. B. PANKO & R. G. SMITH. 1985. Mechanism of androgen-receptor augmentation. Analysis of receptor synthesis and degradation by the density-shift technique. J. Biol. Chem. **260:** 455-461.

38. MACDONALD, R. G., W. C. OKULICZ & W. W. LEAVITT. 1982. Progesterone-induced inactivation of nuclear estrogen receptor in hamster uterus is mediated by acid phosphatase. Biochem. Biophysics Res. Commun. **104:** 570-576.

39. ASTWOOD, E. B. 1939. An assay method for progesterone based upon the decidual cell reaction in the rat. J. Endocrinol. **1:** 49-55.

40. DO, Y. S. & W. W. LEAVITT. 1978. Characterization of a specific progesterone receptor in decidualized hamster uterus. Endocrinology **102:** 443-451.

41. KIMMEL, G. L., B. C. MOULTON & W. W. LEAVITT. 1973. Uptake and retention of [³H] oestradiol by myometrial and deciduomal tissue in the pseudopregnant rat. J. Endocrinol. **56:** 335-336.

42. TALLEY, D. J., J. A. TOBERT, E. G. ARMSTRONG & C. A. VILLEE. 1977. Changes in estrogen receptor levels during deciduomata development in the pseudopregnant rat. Endocrinology **101:** 1538-1544.

43. PELEG, S., S. BAUMINGER & H. R. LINDER. 1979. Oestrogen and progestin receptors in deciduoma of the rat. J. Steroid Biochem. **10:** 139-145.

44. MOULTON, B. C. & B. B. KOENIG. 1981. Estrogen receptor in deciduoma cells separated by velocity sedimentation. Endocrinology **108:** 484-490.

Macrophages and Implantation

CHIKASHI TACHI[a,c] AND SUMIE TACHI[b]

[a]Zoological Institute
Faculty of Science
University of Tokyo, Bunkyo-ku
Tokyo 113, Japan

[b]Department of Anatomy
Tokyo Women's Medical College
Ichigaya-Kawada-cho
Shinjuku-ku, Tokyo 162, Japan

INTRODUCTION

The remarkable complexity of the mechanisms that underlie the immunological peculiarities of the fetomaternal relationship in eutherian mammals has gradually been unveiled in the past three decades. A crucial gap of knowledge remains yet to be filled, however, in order to sufficiently explain the enigmatic condition of true viviparity.

Particularly in need of clarification are the factors responsible for controlling the afferent flow of immunological information from the embryo to the maternal immune system during the perinidatory period of gestation. The regulated flow of the immunological information during that period will be one of the most critical events throughout the entire course of pregnancy from the viewpoint of establishing immunological embryo-maternal relationships. In order to approach the problem, it will be essential to investigate and characterize the nature of immune responses that take place locally in the endometrium during implantation.

Lobel et al.[1-3] made detailed histological analyses of the implantation sites in the rat endometrium and described the distribution of neutrophils, eosinophils, and lymphocytes in the region. Their studies, however, were limited to qualitative assessment of the sectioned specimens observed at light microscopic levels. Furthermore, macrophages were not included in their study except for brief mention of monocytes infiltrating the surface endometrium during the early postnidatory period.[1]

In fact, surprisingly little attention has been paid to the role played by macrophages during nidation until relatively recently (C. Tachi et al.[4]), despite

[c]One of the authors (C. Tachi) gratefully acknowledges the financial support given to him from the Rockefeller Foundation, New York, NY, which enabled him to attend the Symposium.

the fact that they are one of the most versatile and crucial members of the immunological defence mechanism of the mammalian body.

We carried out a series of experiments in order to understand the mechanisms underlying local immune responses during nidation in the Muridae rodents, with special reference to macrophages.[4-8] The results so far obtained will be summarized and presented as a review in this paper.

XENOGENEIC IMPLANTATION OF RAT (RATTUS NORVEGICUS) BLASTOCYSTS ONTO THE ENDOMETRIUM OF THE MOUSE (MUS MUSCULUS)

Our interests in the possible role played by macrophages during nidation were aroused while we were working on the problems of experimentally induced implantation of rat blastocysts onto the endometrium of the mouse (S. Tachi and C. Tachi).[9] The series of experiments was planned with the expectation that the xenogeneic embryos, being highly immunogenic to the host, might disturb the mechanisms responsible for the protection of the conceptuses during gestation, and that the analysis of the fate of the xenogeneic implants might provide us with clues necessary for the elucidation of the immunological mechanisms underlying the natural allogeneic pregnancy.

Experimental transfer of rat blastocysts to the uterus of the mouse was originally attempted by Briones and Beatty.[10] The experiments were repeated later by Tarkowski[11] and by Potts et al.[12] Considerable disparity, however, existed among the results reported by the different authors.

According to the observations made by Briones and Beatty,[10] the rat embryos survived but did neither develop nor implant in the uterus of the pseudopregnant mouse during the period of 24-48 hr after transfer. On the other hand, Tarkowski[11] observed, following similar transfer experiments, that rat blastocysts successfully completed the seemingly normal attachment reactions to the luminal epithelium of the mouse uterus, although none of the implants could survive beyond four days after transfer.

Potts et al.[12] attempted to analyze at ultrastructural levels the interactions between the rat blastocysts and the luminal epithelium of the mouse uterus following the intergeneric embryo transfer. They concluded that the trophoblast cells of the transferred rat embryos were unable to establish firm cellular contact with the luminal epithelium of the mouse uterus during the initial stage of implantation.

Among the three different groups of investigators who made independent attempts on the experimental transfer of rat blastocysts to the uterus of the mouse, only Tarkowski[11] reported the successful occurrence of the xenogeneic implantation. His observations, however, were made at light microscopic levels, and no further analysis of the phenomenon was attempted.

We therefore decided to make an independent attempt to transfer rat blastocysts to the mouse uterus, and if the embryos were indeed capable of accomplishing nidation, then we would analyze the process at ultrastructural levels. We used as the host either normal mice (S. Tachi and C. Tachi[9]) or nude mice (nu/nu) that, congenitally lacking the thymus, are defunct in T-cell mediated immunity and capable of successfully taking wide variety of xenogeneic transplants (C. Tachi et al.[13]) The results obtained are summarized below.

Throughout the following accounts, the day on the morning of which either spermatozoa in the vaginal smear or a copulatory plug was found was designated day 1 of gestation in rats as well as in mice.

Normal Mouse as the Host

Rat blastocysts were collected around noon on day 5 of pregnancy and transferred to the uterus of the mouse on day 3. Altogether 430 rat blastocysts were transferred and 37 were recovered as implants. None of the transferred blastocysts, however, was found surviving in the mouse uterus beyond 96 hrs after transfer (TABLE 1). Our results confirmed the observations made by Tarkowski,[11] but differed from those reported by Briones and Beatty[10] or by Potts et al.[12]

Electron microscopic observation of the recovered implantation sites revealed that the xenogenic implants successfully undergo the early attachment stage and the late attachment stage of implantation (S. Tachi and C. Tachi[9]). The foreign implants, however, invariably degenerated shortly after the onset of the invasion stage. The results of our observations are summarized as a schematic drawing in FIGURE 1.

Nude Mouse as the Host

Experimental transfer of rat blastocysts to the uteri of nude mice with expectation that the foreign embryos might survive better in the uteri of the immunodeficient mutant mice was carried out by Håkansson et al.[13] and by ourselves (C. Tachi;[14] and C. Tachi et al.[15]).

We transferred a total of 295 rat blastocysts to the uterus of pseudopregnant nude mice and recovered 15 xenogeneic implants.[15] No implants, however, were found surviving in the host uteri 96 hrs after transfer (TABLE 2). Our results basically agreed with those reported by Håkansson et al.[13] They noted, however, that the rat blastocysts transferred to the nude mice outlived those in heterozygous controls by approximately three days,[13] whereas we found that the xenogeneic implants degenerated in the uterus of nude mice at approximately the same time as in either the normal or the heterozygous control mice.[14,15]

In short, the uterine environment of nude mice does not provide any

TABLE 1. Implantation of Rat Blastocysts in The Uterus of The Mouse[9]

Time of killing in hour after transfer	Approximate age of rat blastocysts at time of killing	Number of rat blastocysts transferred	Number of recipient mice	Number of successful implantation sites recovered	Number of decidual nodules without implants
36	144 hr pc[a]	17	3	2	0
48	156 hr pc	85	10	4	0
52	160 hr pc	49	5	11	1
56	164 hr pc	134	12	11	7
72	180 hr pc	98	10	9	17
96	204 hr pc	33	4	0	8
120	228 hr pc	14	3	0	1
Total		430	47	37	34

[a] pc = post coitum

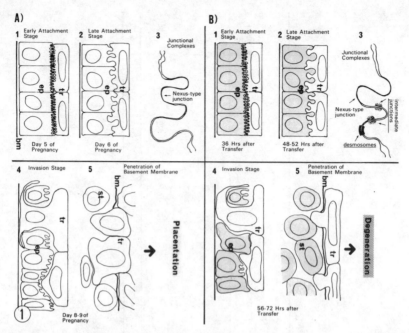

FIGURE 1. Schematic drawings illustrating the ultrastructural processes of the normal allogeneic and experimentally induced xenogeneic implantation of rat blastocysts. **A:** Allogeneic implantation (rat blastocyst onto the rat endometrium). **B:** Xenogeneic implantation (rat blastocyst onto the mouse endometrium).

significantly better environment for the survival of rat blastocysts than that of normal mice. The results strongly indicated to us, that the T-cell mediated cellular immunity of the host might not play any essential role in the degeneration of the xenogeneic implants in the uterus of the mouse.

TRANSPLANTATION OF RAT TROPHOBLASTIC TISSUES TO NUDE MICE

On the basis of the foregoing results, we decided to examine the fate of rat trophoblastic tissues transplanted to various sites in the nude mice (C. Tachi et al.[15]). Trophoblastic tissues from the ectoplacental cone, where trophoblast cells undergo active proliferation, were used for this purpose.

Contrary to our original expectation, the rat trophoblastic tissues transplanted subcutaneously to the nude mice regressed approximately at the same rate as those transplanted to the control mice (nu/+).[15] We carried out similar experiments with different combinations of conditions of hosts and/

or sites of transplantation (TABLE 3). The transplants invariably degenerted by the time of the examination except in the group of nude mice that had been treated with carrageenan, a potent inhibitor of macrophage activities. Those results led us to examine the possibility that macrophages might be involved in the early maternal responses to the implantation.

Because macrophages are responsible for the primary processing of immunogens and for transmitting the information to T cells, it is conceivable that they might play a crucial role as one of the most significant elements of the afferent arm of the embryo-maternal relationships during the perinidatory period of gestation.

MACROPHAGES IN THE POSTNIDATORY UTERUS OF THE RAT

In order to demonstrate macrophages in the uterine tissues during the early gestation, the classical India ink method was chosen. This method is one of the oldest ones devised for the demonstration of macrophages in histological specimens of animal tissues. Despite the many shortcomings and possible pitfalls that one must pay attention to in interpreting the results, the method is used today as one of the standard techniques for the purpose.

A solution of India ink was injected into a tail vein of the rats on different days of reproductive cycles, and the animals were killed 12-24 hrs afterwards (TABLE 4) (C. Tachi et al.[4]). The implantation sites were fixed, sectioned, and stained with hematoxylin and eosin according to the procedures commonly employed for histological observations by light microscopy. Examination of the specimens revealed that the numerous phagocytes loaded with carbon particles were present around the nidus shortly after the onset of implantation. Such phagocytes, however, were curiously absent within the decidua (FIG. 2).

Most of those phagocytes were ascertained to be macrophages on account of the following experimental findings.

1) When the frozen sections of the rat uterus collected during the perinidatory period of gestation were histochemically stained for the presence of nonspecific esterase that had been used as a marker enzyme of macrophages,

TABLE 2. Implantation of Rat Blastocysts in the Uterus of the Nude Mouse[15]

Time of killing (hr)	Approximate age of blastocysts at time of killing (hr post coitum)	Number of blastocysts transferred	Number of successful implantation sites
48	85	32	3
72	180	206	12
92	200	57	0
Total		295	15

TABLE 3. Survival of the Trophoblastic Tissues Ectopically Transplanted to Homozygous (nu/nu) or Heterozygous (nu/+) nude mice. (C. Tachi & M. Yokoyama, unpublished).

Animals and treatment	Sources of trophoblastic tissues	Sites of transplantation	Time of killing in days after transplantation	Number of animals used	Number of animals with transplants at autopsy
nu/nu	BLC	kidney capsule	14	10	2
nu/+	BLC	kidney capsule	14	10	3
nu/nu	EPC	kidney capsule	20	6	0
nu/+	EPC	kidney capsule	20	8	0
nu/nu	EPC	subcutaneous	20	5	0
nu/+	EPC	subcutaneous	20	5	0
nu/nu + PMS hCG[a]	EPC	subcutaneous	20	6	4 (trace)
nu/nu	EPC	intraperitoneal	7[c]	5	1
nu/nu +CGN 4 mg[b]	EPC	intraperitoneal	7	5	4 (infection)
nu/nu +CGN 20 mg	EPC	intraperitoneal	7	4	4 (infection)

[a] Pregnant mare's serum gonadotropin (PMS) was injected at a dose level of 10 IU/mouse. Human chorionic gonadotropin (hCG, 10 IU/mouse) was injected 48 hrs afterwards. Both injections were made intraperitoneally (i.p.). Transplantation was carried out approximately 24 hrs after the injection of hCG.

[b] Carrageenan (CGN) was suspended in saline at a concentration of 40 mg/ml. Immediately after the surgery, 0.1 ml or 0.5 ml of the suspension was administered i.p. to the animals of the 4 mg or 20 mg group respectively.

[c] The time course of the diappearance of the transplanted tissues partly depends upon the initial amount of the tissues transplanted. In our experiments, most of the tissues regressed almost entirely by one week after the transplantation (see ref. 15). In this group of the experiments, the animals were killed earlier than those of the other groups because of the severe bacterial infection that affected the CGN-treated animals.

cells intensely stained with the dye were found in the endometrial stroma. Furthermore, the patterns of the distribution of such cells were strikingly similar to that of the phagocytes loaded with carbon particles; the cells carrying nonspecific esterase at a high concentration were numerously found around but not within the decidua (FIG. 3) (C. Tachi et al.[4]).

2) Ultrastructural characteristics of the carbon-loaded phagocytes coincided well with those generally attributed to macrophages (C. Tachi et al.[4]).

3) Yeast glucan that had been known as the activator of macrophage activities in vivo when administered by injection to animals[17,18] seemingly intensified the uptake of the carbon particles by the phagocytes present near the implantation site (C. Tachi, in preparation).

When the postnidatory uteri of the rats treated with India ink were fixed and cleared with xylene, the implantation sites were clearly visible as the

TABLE 4. Schedule of Treatment[a] of the Animals for the Demonstration of Macrophages in the Endometrium during Early Gestation[4]

			D_1	D_2	D_3	D_4	D_5	D_6	D_7
Pregnancy	D1	3	■—▲						
	D2	3		■—▲					
	D3	3			■—▲				
	D4	3				■—▲			
	D5-A	3					■—▲		
	D5-B	3					■—▲		
	D5-C	3						■—▲	
	D6	3						■—▲	

[a] Dotted line and broken line represent noon and midnight respectively. Solid square = time when India ink was injected; solid triangle = time when the animals were killed; $D_1 - D_7$ = day of pregnancy.

blackened areas. The blackening was more intense in the antimesometrial region than in the mesometrial region.

Psychoyos[19] originally described the increase in capillary permeability as one of the earliest endometrial responses taking place after the onset of implantation. He administered intravenously a solution of macromolecular dye, Geigy blue, to rats during the perinidatory period, and observed that the "blueing reactions," due to the leakage of the dye from capillaries, take place at the implantation sites that are not recognizable by other means.

In FIGURE 4, two sets of the uteri with the "blackening" reactions are shown. The two uterine horns on the left are those from the control rats that received the injection of India ink solution only. The other two uterine horns on the right are from the experimental group where the animals were given

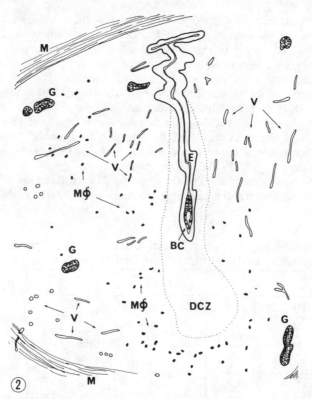

FIGURE 2. Tracing of a photomicrograph of a uterine cross section illustrating the distribution of phagocytic cells near the implantation sites. The phagocytic cells that are loaded with carbon particles of India ink are probably macrophages and encountered particularly frequently around the decidua in the antimesometrial region. BC = blastocyst; DCZ = decidual zone; G = gland; M = myometrium; Mo = macrophages; V = blood vessels. (C. Tachi.[6] With permission from *Zoological Science.*)

FIGURE 3. Histochemical demonstration of the cells with high activity of nonspecific esterase near the implantation site. The specimen was obtained around midnight on day 5 of pregnancy. The cryostat section was stained with pararosaniline according to the method described by Koski *et al.*[16] The cells with the enzymatic activity were stained red. Methyl green was used as a counterstain. The edge of the decidual zone that is stained more heavily than the nondecidualized endometrial stroma is demarcated by arrow heads. The luminal and glandular epithelial cells reacted positively to the dye. In the endometrial stroma, cells stained heavily with the dye appeared in clusters of several cells around the decidual zone. Few cells with the positive reaction, however, appeared in the decidual zone. DCZ = decidual zone; L = luminal epithelium; G = glandular epithelium. (C. Tachi *et al.*[4] With permission from the *Journal of Experimental Zoology.*)

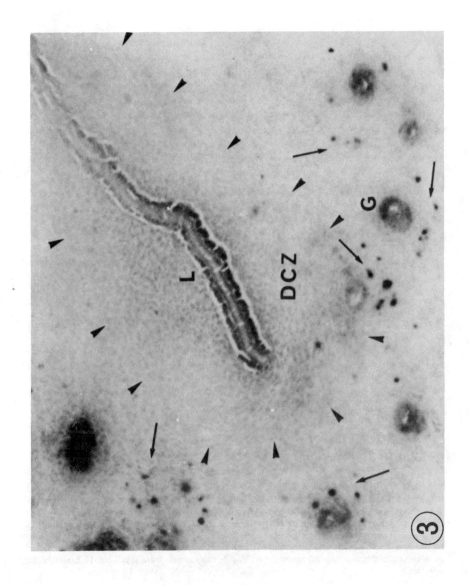

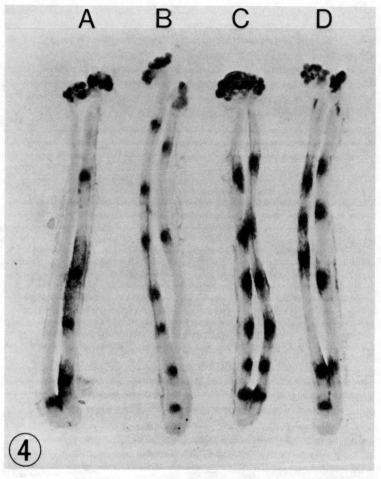

FIGURE 4. "Blackening reactions" in the postnidatory uteri following a single intravenous injection of India ink solution given at midnight of day 5. The animals were killed at noon of day 6, that is, 12 hrs after the injection. A) and B), uteri of the control rats. C) and D), uteri from rats of the experimental group where the animals were pretreated with daily injections of yeast glucan suspended in saline at a concentration of 5 mg/ml, from day 2 until day 4. Two ml of the solution was injected intravenously into a tail vein. India ink solution was administered as in the control group around midnight on day 5; the animals were sacrificed 12 hrs after the injection.

daily injections of yeast glucan suspended in saline, from day 2 until day 4. The animals of both the experimental and the control groups received the injection of India ink on day 5. As clearly seen in the figure, the blackening reactions in the animals belonging to the experimental group are much stronger than those in the control group. The results indicate that either the activities or the number of the phagocytes that were present around the implantation sites and took up the extravasated carbon particles had increased following treatment with the yeast glucan.

All the experimental evidence we obtained so far does not contradict the assumption that the phagocytes loaded with the carbon particles and found near the implantation sites in the postnidatory endometrium are macrophages. On account of these findings, we tentatively concluded that the macrophages are involved in the early maternal responses to the implantation of blastocysts and that the decidua might act as a barrier against migration of macrophages toward the embryos during the initial stages of nidation (C. Tachi et al.[4]).

In the experiments described so far, we used rats as our material. In order to carry out further analyses of the role played by macrophages during nidation, however, mice are obviously more suitable material than rats, because the former are better understood either immunologically or genetically than the latter.

DISTRIBUTION OF IMMUNOCYTES THAT BIND IMMUNOGLOBULINS IN THE POSTNIDATORY UTERUS OF THE MOUSE

The macrophages demonstrated in the endometrium by their nonimmune mediated phagocytic activities are not representative of the entire population of the macrophages in the tissue. Furthermore, immunocytes other than macrophages are probably involved in the early local immune responses in the endometrium to the implantation. Therefore, as an initial approach to the problems, we analyzed the distribution of immunocytes that carry different species of immunoglobulins as a cellular marker in the uterus of the mouse during postnidatory period of gestation (C. Tachi et al.[6]). Frozen sections of the implantation sites of the mouse were cut on a cryostat; they were fixed with 90% ethanol and stained with FITC-labeled anti-IgG antibodies.

FIGURE 5 shows that fluorescein-labeled cells in the specimen collected around 1600 on day 5 of pregnancy. The labeled cells were found in the endometrial stroma (FIG. 5), in the myometrium (FIG. 5), and in the mesometrial triangle (FIG. 5) (C. Tachi[6]). The labeled cells were scarcely found in the luminal as well as the glandular epithelium of the endometrium. The lumens of the glands were faintly stained, indicating the presence of IgG in the secretion products of the glands (FIG. 5). In the myometrium, numerous FITC-labeled cells were seen in the connective tissues located between the longitudinal and the circular muscular layers. Their distribution appeared to be in close association with the blood vessels (FIG. 5). Essentially similar

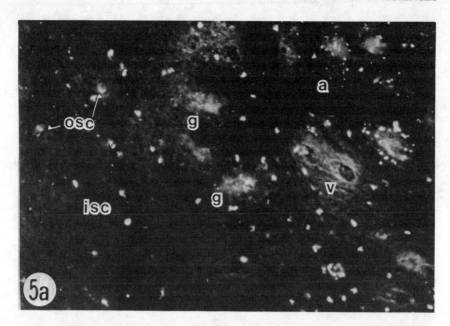

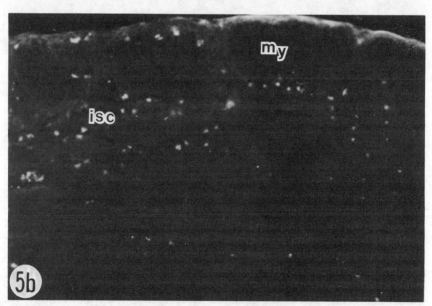

FIGURE 5a-c. Cells binding FITC-labeled anti-IgG antibodies in different areas of a cross section of a gestational uterus cut through the implantation site. The animal was killed around 1600 on day 5 of pregnancy. **a:** Endometrial stroma; **b:** myometrium, and **c:** mesometrial triangle. a = autofluorescent material; v = blood vessels; g = gland; isc = intensely stained small cells; osc = oval shaped cells; mt = mesometrial triangle; my = myometrium. (C. Tachi.[6] With permission from Zoological Science.)

observations were made in the uterine specimens collected on day 6 and day 7 of gestation.

The FITC-labeled cells observed in the uterus during the early period of gestation ranging from day 5 to day 7 were grossly classified into two types. The cells belonging to the first type were small in size and round in shape and were intensely stained with FITC-labeled antibodies. The majority of the labeled cells were of this type (FIG. 5).

The cells of the second type were oval shaped; they were larger in size than those of the first type and only occasionally encountered (FIG. 5a and c). They were often found in the vicinity of the gland (FIG. 5a) and in the mesometrial triangle where they were seen forming a small cluster consisting of several cells (FIG. 5c).

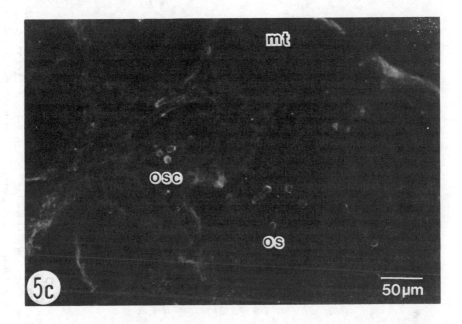

The lack of the FITC-labeled cells within the decidual zones formed around the conceptuses is one of the salient observations made in this series of the experiments. In FIGURE 6, the tracings of photomicrographs are presented showing the distribution of FITC-labeled cells in representative cross sections of implantation sites collected on day 5, day 6, and day 7 (C. Tachi et al.[4]).

The results of the quantitative evaluation of the distribution of the FITC-labeled cells in the cross section of the day 7 uterus is shown in FIGURE 7. In this specimen, less than 3% of the entire FITC-labeled cell population were found in the decidual area. It also can be seen in the figure that more labeled cells were present in the antimesometrial area than in the mesometrial

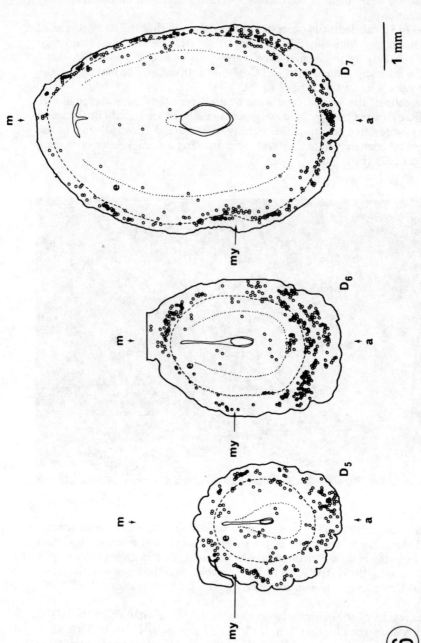

FIGURE 6. Tracings of photomicrographs of uterine cross sections illustrating the distribution of the FITC-labeled cells. The positions of the labeled cells were marked with small circles in the figure. The decidual zone is demarcated by fine dotted lines. Tracings were made on enlarged photomicrographs by means of a computer-aided graphic analysis system in our laboratory. The software used, TACSYS/G (ver 4.0), was originally written for the system by one of the present authors (C. Tachi). Some of those fluorescent spots that could be only dubiously identified as cells were inevitably included in the figure. a = antimesometrial side; m = mesometrial side; e = endometrium; my = myometrium. (C. Tachi et al.[4] With permission from the *Journal of Experimental Zoology*).

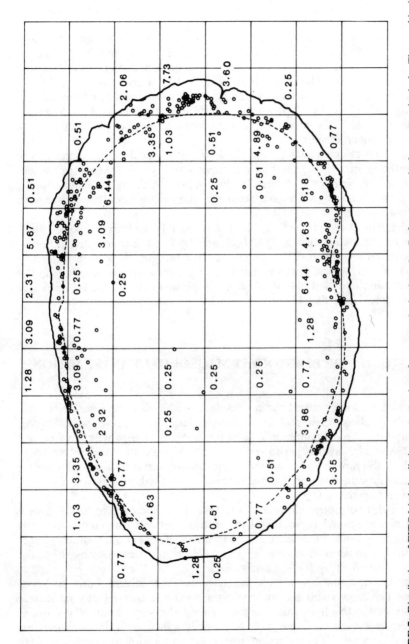

FIGURE 7. Distribution of FITC-labeled cells in a cross section of a uterus obtained on day 7 of pregnancy is shown quantitatively. The graphic data were processed by using TACSYS/G(ver. 4) as described in the legend for FIGURE 6. Numerical figures in each square indicate (in percent) the relative number of FITC-labeled cells found within the area. (C. Tachi.[6] With permission from *Zoological Science*.)

area, that is, approximately 48% in the former and 22% in the latter. The result is typical of many others obtained by analyzing specimens collected on day 7 and processed similarly.

We carried out similar experiments using FITC-labeled anti-IgA, and anti-IgE antibodies. Anti-IgA antibodies stained the glandular lumen intensely. The myometrium of the uterus also gave a strong reaction to the antibodies (FIG. 8). The distribution of cells that binds anti-IgA in the implantation sites was remarkably similar to that obtained for the anti-IgG binding cells (FIG. 8). Experiments where anti-IgE was used gave similar results, and the FITC-labeled cells were found in the periphery of decidua and in the myometrium.

Lobel et al.[2] concluded, as a result of histological observations of the implantation sites in the rat, that eosinophils and lymphocytes were concentrated at the periphery of the decidual nodes. Although no quantitative analysis was done by them, our results in the mouse essentially agree with their observations.

Rachman et al.[20] as well as M. B. Parr and E. L. Parr[21] reported their results on the localization of IgA, IgG, and IgM in the endometrium during the perinidatory period. They concluded that IgA and IgG were located in plasma cells in the endometrium surrounding uterine glands as well as in the gland lumina and that the number of the plasma cells increased markedly between day 1 and day 4.

EM STUDIES OF BLASTOCYST-MACROPHAGE INTERACTIONS

In order to understand the mechanisms underlying the interactions between trophoblast cells and immunocytes, including macrophages during implantation, the examination of such interactions in vitro will be of value.

Glass et al.[23] layered peritoneal macrophages onto the trophoblastic outgrowth of the mouse and concluded that the free surfaces of the trophoblast cells are not adhesive for the macrophages. No further analyses, however, were made by the authors.

We cultured mouse blastocysts together with macrophages of allogeneic origin and examined the mode of interactions between the embryonic cells and the phagocytes of ultrastructural levels (S. Tachi et al.[8]). Macrophages used for the experiments were collected as peritoneal exudate by using the methods described by Knyszynski et al.[22]

For the first few hours after the initiation of coculture, both the zona-encased blastocysts and the macrophages remained without any noticeable changes under the light microscope. Around the sixth hour of coculture, however, many macrophages were seen firmly adhering to the zona in some of the blastocysts. The adhesion was firm, and those macrophages were removed only after repeated washing of the embryos with fresh medium (FIG. 9). Many blastocysts shed their zona approximately 26 hrs after the start of

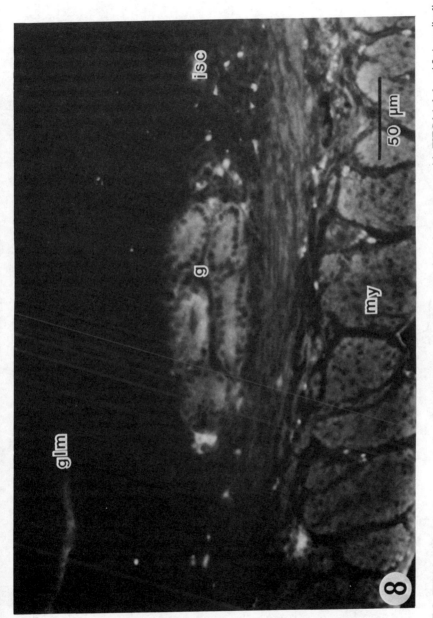

FIGURE 8. FITC-labeled cells in a cross section of uterus on day 6 of pregnancy following treatment with FITC-labeled anti-IgA antibodies. The figure pictures a cross section of a gestational uterus. The animal was killed around 1600 on day 5 of pregnancy. Preparation of the cryostat sections and staining with the fluorescein labeled anti-IgA antibodies were carried out as described previously.[6] g = gland; glm = glandular lumen; isc = intensely stained small cells; my = myometrium.

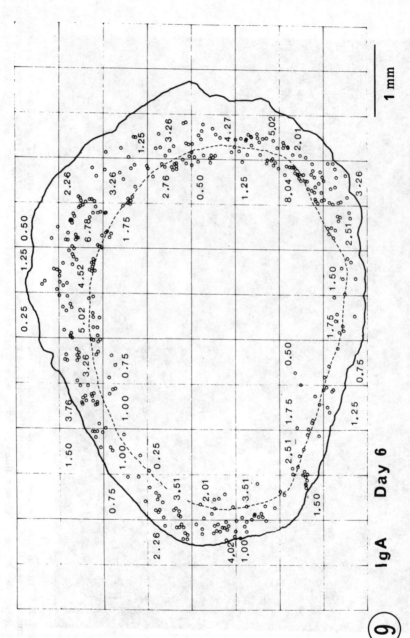

FIGURE 9. Distribution of the cells that bound FITC-labeled anti-IgA antibodies in a cross section of uterus obtained on day 6 of pregnancy. The animal was killed around noon of day 6. Cryostat sections were treated with the fluorescein-labeled antibodies as described previously.[6] The tracing of the photomicrographs and the evaluation of the relative densities of the labeled cells were carried out as described in the legend for FIGURE 6.

coculture. The macrophages had adhered to the surface of the zona as well as to the exposed surfaces of the trophoblast cells.

Although many macrophages were present on the empty zonae pellucidae shed by the blastocysts that remained in the culture, the surfaces of the hatched embryos were relatively free from the phagocytes. The majority of the blastocysts were without their zona by the 48th hour of coculture, and had attached to the bottom surfaces of the culture dishes. Trophoblastic spreading had been initiated in many of such blastocysts.

At the periphery of the trophoblastic outgrowth, signs of neither accu-

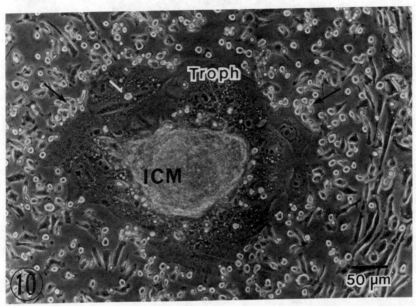

FIGURE 10. A blastocyst undergoing trophoblastic spreading approximately 48 hrs after the initiation of coculture. A well-developed ICM is seen in the center of the embryo. Macrophages (black arrows) appear to have been physically pushed aside by the growing trophoblast cells. Several macrophages (white arrow) are present on the surface of the spreading trophoblast cells. (S. Tachi & C. Tachi.[8] With permission from *Zoological Science.*)

mulation nor repulsion of macrophages were apparent (FIG. 10). Often, macrophages were observed within the trophoblast cell layer during this period; they tended to be localized around the inner cell mass (ICM) (FIG. 10).

The interface between the trophoblast cell layer and the macrophages was examined electron microscopically (FIG. 11). The trophoblast cells in the region extended cytoplasmic processes that were 0.5-1.4 μm in thickness and contained cytoplasmic filaments, endoplasmic reticulum, and mitochondria (FIG. 11). The cytoplasmic processes were often in contact with macrophages as if they were pushing aside the phagocytes with physical force (FIG. 11).

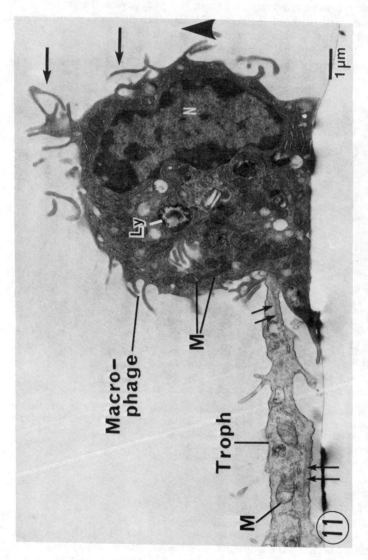

FIGURE 11. Electron micrograph showing a trophoblast cell in contact with a macrophage at the periphery of the trophoblastic outgrowth in the 48th hr of coculture. The macrophage is slightly tilted as if it is physically pushed by the cytoplasmic process extended by the trophoblast cell. Note the difference in the size of mitochondria in the trophoblast cell and those in the macrophage. Ly = lysosome; M = mitochondria; N = nucleus; Troph = trophoblast cell. Thick arrows = cytoplasmic processes of macrophage; double arrows = thin filaments. (S. Tachi & C. Tachi.[8] With permission from *Zoological Science*.).

The macrophages, on the other hand, possessed many long and irregularly shaped villous projections extended from their surfaces; the cytoplasm was electron dense and contained lysosomes, rough-surfaced endoplasmic reticula, and mitochondria (FIG. 11). Around the 72d hr of coculture, macrophages were present not only on the surfaces of the trophoblast cells but also inside the embryos.

The macrophages in the embryos were completely enclosed by the trophoblast cells and ICM cells (FIG. 12). Close contact is formed between the macrophages and ICM cells, and in some specimens the formation of desmosomes at the junctions was confirmed.

Occasionally, debris of the phagocytized cells was observed in the cytoplasm of the trophoblast cells observed during this period. Although it was not possible to definitely identify the type of the ingested cells, they were probably macrophages.

On the fourth day of coculture, an outermost layer of the ICM cells comprised the primitive endoderm cells that were covered with numerous microvilli and characterized by the presence of large vacuoles in the peripheral area of their cytoplasm covered with numerous microvilli on their surfaces. Macrophages were often seen adhering to the primitive endoderm cells. The site of contact between a cytoplasmic process extended by a macrophage and the cell membrane of an endodermal cell is shown at a high magnification in FIGURE 8.

Under the experimental conditions we employed, the ICM cells of the cultured blastocysts had invariably degenerated by the fifth day of culture regardless of the presence or the absence of macrophages. Therefore, it was impossible to definitely ascertain whether the macrophages were cytotoxic to the ICM cells or not.

It was surprising for us that trophoblast cells that behaved as active phagocytes toward the luminal epithelial cells of the endometrium during the invasion stage of implantation[24] exhibited neither explicit cytotoxicity nor strong phagocytic activities toward the macrophages in culture. The majority of macrophages appeared to have been simply pushed aside physically during the course of trophoblastic spreading. Although occasional phagocytosis of cells by the trophoblast cells were observed on the fourth day of coculture, no quantitative analysis of this phenomenon was attempted in the present series of the experiments.

CONCLUSIONS

Many questions remain to be answered concerning the roles played by macrophages during implantation. What activates macrophages during early gestation? Why and how does the decidua act as a barrier? Does the control of local immune responses during early gestation provide a means for fertility control? What are the causes for incompatibility between embryos and the

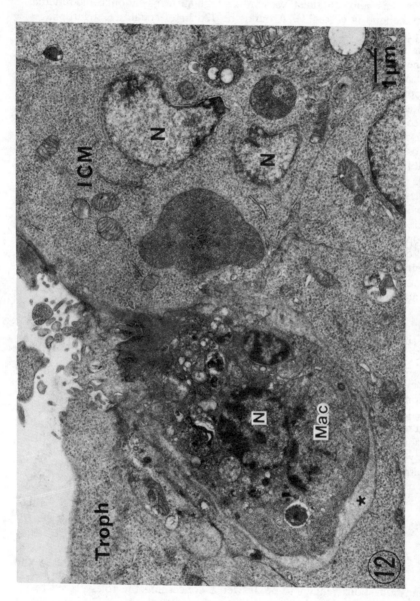

FIGURE 12. Electron micrograph showing a macrophage found in the cultured blastocyst around the 72d hr of coculture. The macrophage is completely surrounded by trophoblast cells and an ICM cell. The space (*) between the macrophage and the trophoblast cells is filled with an amorphous substance of moderate electron density. ICM = inner cell mass cells; Mac = macrophage; N = nucleus; Troph = trophoblast cells. (S. Tachi & C. Tachi.[8] With permission from *Zoological Science.*)

mother following xenogeneic implantation in Muridae rodents? Do the local immune responses following implantation of transgenic embryos act as a cause for the transmission distortion of the foreign genetic information? Experiments are in progress in our laboratory to help answer, at least in part, some of these questions.

REFERENCES

1. LOBEL, B. L., E. LEVY & M. C. SHELESNYAK. 1967. Studies on the mechanisms of nidation. XXXIV. Dynamics of cellular interactions during progestation and implantation in the rat. Part II. Nidus formation. Acta Endocrinol. suppl. **123:** 47-75.

2. LOBEL, B. L., E. LEVY & M. C. SHELESNYAK. 1967. Studies on the mechanisms of nidation. XXXIV. Dynamics of cellular interactions during progestation and implantation in the rat. Part III. Implantation. Acta Endocrinol. suppl. **123:** 77-109.

3. LOBEL, B. L., E. LEVY, E. S. KISCH & M. C. SHELESNYAK. 1967. Studies on the mechanisms of nidation. XXVIII. Experimental investigation on the origin of eosinophilic granulocytes in the uterus of the rat. Acta Endocrinol. **55:** 451-457.

4. TACHI, C., S. TACHI & H. R. LINDNER. 1981. Possible involvement of macrophages in embryo-maternal relationships during ovum implantation in the rat. J. Exp. Zool. **217:** 81-92.

5. TACHI, C. 1983. Analysis of local immune responses during implantation in the mouse. (Abstract in Japanese). Zoological Magazine **92:** 505.

6. TACHI, C. 1985. Mechanisms underlying regulation of local immune responses in the uterus during early gestation of eutherian mammals. I. Distribution of immuno-competent cells which bind anti-IgG antibodies in the post-nidatory uterus of the mouse. Zool. Sci., **2:** 341-348.

7. TACHI, S. & C. TACHI. 1981. Interactions between blastocysts and macrophages *in vitro*. (Abstract). Acta Anat. Nippon. **56:** 241-242.

8. TACHI, S. & C. TACHI. 1985. Mechanisms underlying regulation of local immune responses in the uterus during early gestation of eutherian mammals. II. Electron microscopic studies in the interactions between blastocysts and macrophages cultured together *in vitro*. Zool. Sci. **2:** 671-680.

9. TACHI, S. & C. TACHI. 1979. Ultrastructural studies on maternal-embryonic cell interaction during experimentally induced implantation of rat blastocysts to the endometrium of the mouse. Dev. Biol. **68:** 203-223.

10. BRIONES, H. & R. A. BEATTY. 1954. Inter-specific transfers of rodent eggs. J. Exp. Zool. **125:** 99-118.

11. TARKOWSKI, A. K. 1962. Interspecific transfers of eggs between rat and mouse. J. Embryol. Exp. Morphol. **10,** 476-495.

12. POTTS, D. M., I. B. WILSON & M. S. R. SMITH. 1970. Observations on rat eggs transplanted to the mouse uterus. J. Reprod. Fertil. **22:** 425-428.

13. HÅKANSSON, S., O. LUNDKVIST, O. NILSSON & G. ALM. 1977. Prolonged survival of implanting rat blastocysts in the uterus of congenitally athymic mice. Scand. J. Immunol. **6:** 817-820.

14. TACHI, C. 1977. Implantation of rat blastocysts xenogeneically transferred to the uterus of nude mouse. *In* Scientific Report of the Research Project on Nude Mice Sponsored by the Science & Technology Agency of Japan. (Abstract in Japanese). p. 22.

15. TACHI, C., S. TACHI, M. YOKOYAMA & N. OSAWA. 1981. Survival of rat blastocysts in the uterus of the mouse following xenogeneic implantation. *In* Cellular and Molecular Aspects of Implantation. S. Glasser & D. W. Bullock, Eds.: 473-475. Plenum Press. New York.

16. KOSKI, I. R., D. G. POPLACK & R. M. BLEASE. 1976. A non-specific esterase stain for the identification of monocytes and macrophage. *In In vitro* Methods in Cell-Mediated and Tumour Immunity. B. R. Bloom & J. R. David, Eds.: 359-362. Academic Press. New York.
17. BURGALETA, C., M. C. TORRITO, S. G. QUAN & D. W. GOLDE. 1978. Glucan activated macrophages : functional characteristics and surface morphology. J. Reticuloendothelial Soc. Med. **23**: 195-211.
18. DI LUZIO, N. R. 1979. Lysozyme, glucan-activated macrophages and neoplasia. J. Reticuloendothelial Soc. Med. **26**: 67-81.
19. PSYCHOYOS, A. 1960. La réaction déciduale est précédée de modifications précoces de la perméabilite capillaire de l'utérus. C. R. Soc. Biol. **154**: 1384-1387.
20. RACHMAN, F., V. CASIMIRI & O. BERNARD. 1984. Maternal immunoglobulins G, A and M in mouse uterus and embryo during the postimplantation period. J. Reprod. Immunol. **6**: 39-47.
21. PARR, M. B. & E. L. PARR. 1985. Immunohistochemical localization of immunoglobulins A, G, and M in the mouse female genital tract. J. Reprod. Fertil. **74**: 361-370.
22. KNYSZYNSKI, A., S. J. LEIBOVICH & D. DANON. 1977. Phagocytosis of "old" red blood cells by macrophages from syngeneic mice *in vitro*. Exp. Hemat. **5**: 480-486.
23. GLASS, R. H., A. I. SPINDLE, M. MAGLIO & R. A. PEDERSEN. 1980. The free surface of mouse trophoblast in culture is non-adhesive for other cells. J. Reprod. Fertil. **59**: 403-407.
24. TACHI, S., C. TACHI & H. R. LINDNER. 1970. Ultrastructural features of blastocyst attachment and trophoblastic invasion in the rat. J. Reprod. Fertil. **21**: 37-56.

Immunological Role of the Cellular Constituents of the Decidua in the Maintenance of Semiallogeneic Pregnancy[a]

PEEYUSH K. LALA, MARY KEARNS,[b] RANJIT S.
PARHAR, JOHN SCODRAS, AND SIGRID JOHNSON

Department of Anatomy
The University of Western Ontario
London, Ontario, Canada N6A 5C1

It is indeed a great honor for us to be invited to contribute to this International Symposium on nidation in tribute to Professor M. C. Shelesnyak, whose pioneering work on the physiology of decidualization and its relevance to the success of nidation laid the foundation for further studies by many laboratories. The central role exercised by the decidual tissue for the maintenance of pregnancy in many species is amply illustrated in a number of excellent contributions in this volume from reproductive biologists and endocrinologists. This article will examine the decidual tissue through the eyes of an immunobiologist.

THE CONCEPTUS AS AN ALLOGRAFT

In certain forms of viviparous pregnancy in nature, cells of fetal origin remain exposed to the maternal immune system at the maternal-fetal tissue interface so that the conceptus can be regarded as an allograft on the mother's reproductive tract. Nevertheless, this graft remains unharmed *in situ,* in spite of the fact that the pregnant mother is fully capable of rejecting a heterotopic graft of a genetically identical conceptus,[1] indicating that the mechanisms for protection of the semiallogeneic conceptus must operate locally.[2] Following the pioneering studies by numerous investigators, in particular by Beer and Billingham,[3] immunology of reproduction has now emerged as a major dis-

[a] This work was supported by the Medical Research Council of Canada and the National Cancer Institute of Canada.

[b] Present address: Immunology Branch, National Cancer Institute, NIH, Bethesda, Maryland 20892.

cipline including a strong focus of interest in the mechanisms underlying the survival of the fetoplacental unit resulting from a mating between two genetically disparate partners.[4-7]

Major histocompatibility (MHC) antigens of the class 1 type (H-2 D, K and L in the mouse and HLA-A, B and C in the human) serve as the key recognition molecules on the cell surface of a graft for a self/nonself discrimination by the T lymphocytes of the host. During the development of the murine preimplantation embryo, class 1 MHC antigens are detectable on the outer cells of the late morula and the early blastocyst,[8] but the zona pellucida makes the antigenic sites inaccessible to cells of the maternal immune system, namely, antigen presenting macrophages or lymphocytes, even if such cells were to appear within the uterine lumen. Maternal immune response to foreign antigens expressed on cells artificially introduced into the uterine lumen has indeed been documented.[9] The loss of zona pellucida should theoretically render the preimplantation or the periimplantation blastocyst more vulnerable; however, they remain unharmed. This can be best explained by the observation of a stage-specific disappearance of class 1 MHC antigens from the surface of trophoblast cells of the late blastocyst prior to the loss of zona pellucida.[8] This event may be particularly important for a successful implantation of the heterozygous blastocyst and the early development of the placenta in many species in which trophoblast cells breach the uterine epithelium to expose themselves to the maternal immune cells either in the endometrial stroma or the maternal sinusoids. Interestingly, the story does not end here. Somatic cells of most midgestational embryonic tissues in the mouse express class 1 MHC antigens,[10] but the embryo remains sheltered from the maternal immune system by the placenta. At this time, however, placental trophoblast cells that remain at the fetomaternal interface are no longer antigenically inert. Class 1 MHC antigens of both parental allotypes are reexpressed on a large majority of murine trophoblast cells between day 9 of gestation and term.[11,12] The antigenic sites have been localized *in vivo* on the sinusoidal face of the labyrinth[13] and spongiotrophoblasts[14] at the light microscopic level and on the plasma membrane of these trophoblast populations including that of the sinusoid-lining microvilli at the ultrastructural level,[15] indicating that these sites remain exposed to the maternal blood. The antigenic sites are also exposed to the maternal decidua,[15] which includes many immigrant cells of the immune system.[6] In the human placenta, syncytiotrophoblast cells lining the maternal sinusoids do not express class 1 antigens;[16-18] however, many cytotrophoblast cells in early gestational (first trimester) placentae express these antigens.[17] The antigen-bearing cells have been localized in the extravillous interstitial columns as well as the cytotrophoblast shell embedded in the decidua.[16,19] In addition to histocompatibility antigens potentially alien to the maternal T lymphocytes, trophoblast cells, at least in the mouse midgestational placenta, also express target structures recognized by natural killer lymphocytes[20] that can kill a variety of tumor cells and embryonic cells on first contact. Yet there is no evidence for a harmful cytotoxic response of T lymphocytes or natural killer lymphocytes generated against the trophoblast *in situ*. What may be the reasons?

As we have emphasized earlier, the mechanisms of protection of the semiallogeneic conceptus must be sought locally at the fetomaternal interface. For the survival of the graft to be fail-safe, one would like to postulate that nature would endow the graft itself with unique properties to make this possible.[2] Several such properties can be listed for the trophoblast cells as possibilities, some of which remain to be firmly established. (1) The class 1 MHC antigens on the trophoblast may lack in epitopes recognizable by T cells.[2] This hypothesis has not been tested. Another variation of this hypothesis is the possibility that these antigens, although recognizable by antibodies directed against the monomorphic framework determinants of these molecules, may be truncated or defective in their expression of the allotypic determinants, for example, presenting a deletion of the terminal α_1 domain of the heavy chain.[19] Although this remains as a viable possibility for the human trophoblast,[19] this can be excluded for the mouse trophoblast, which has been shown to express both the paternal and the maternal allotypic determinants.[11–15] Furthermore, even in the case of the human, allotypic determinants of the class 1 MHC antigens have been occasionally detectable on some cytotrophoblasts of the early gestational human placenta (G. Stirrat, personal communication). (2) Trophoblast cells produce immunosuppressor molecules at high local concentrations capable of averting an alloreactive immune response. Of the many products of the trophoblast, one strong candidate is progesterone, which has long been recognized as a potent immunosuppressant capable of blocking the cognitive arm of the alloimmune response.[21] Other immunoactive products of the placenta, the precise cellular source of which have not been established, have been reported to block the cognitive, central, as well as effector arms of the immune responses of lymphocytes.[22] (3) Trophoblast cells appear to possess unique membrane properties,[2] making them highly resistant to the lytic mechanism of various cytotoxic cells. Nevertheless, during the course of normal pregnancy, functionally active maternal cytotoxic cells have not been demonstrable *in situ,* for example, in the decidua.[23,24] Thus it appears that nature does not allow the maternal immune response to proceed to the stage of the generation of functional killer cells.

It is highly likely that the responsibility of abrogating a potentially deleterious immune response against the conceptus is shared by both fetal (trophoblast) as well as maternal cells at the maternal-fetal interface. In this article, we shall demonstrate that the cellular constituents of the decidua, decidual cells in particular, play a key immunoprotective role in the maintenance of pregnancy.

COMPARATIVE ANATOMY OF THE DECIDUAL REACTION: POSSIBLE IMMUNOLOGICAL IMPLICATIONS

The decidual reaction involves the appearance of highly specialized cells (decidual cells) in the progestational endometrium usually in response to the implantation of the blastocyst but can also be induced in the hormone-primed endometrium of certain species with the aid of other stimuli.[25,26] Not all placental mammals exhibit a typical decidual reaction in the pregnant endometrium. It is absent in ungulates including ruminants[27] (having epitheliochorial type placentae[28]), but occurs in carnivores, insectivores, rodents, and anthropoids[27] (having endotheliochorial or hemochorial type placentae[28]). It is interesting to note that in the former case, trophoblast cells of the chorion remain sheltered from the maternal immune system by an essentially intact uterine epithelium, whereas in the latter cases, there is a breaching or destruction of this epithelial barrier resulting in a confrontation of the trophoblast to cells of the maternal immune system either in the endometrial stroma or the blood sinusoids. This correlation can hardly be fortuitous, and possibly implies a protective function of the decidua in preventing a harmful maternal immune response against the alloantigen-bearing trophoblast,[29] a function proposed earlier on the basis of grafting experiments with allogeneic blastocysts[30] or skin.[31] This postulate is also consistent with the finding that the extent of decidualization and trophoblast invasiveness appears to run parallel in numerous species,[32] although primates appear to present an exception.[33] An alternate interpretation of this finding is the possible protective role of the decidua against trophoblastic invasion of the uterus.[32,34] Although these possibilities are not mutually exclusive, current evidence in favor of the first postulate is now strong, as will be discussed later.

CONSTITUENTS OF THE DECIDUAL TISSUE: ORIGIN OF THE DECIDUAL CELLS

Decidual tissue is heterogeneous in composition inclusive of typical (stromal type) decidual cells, immigrant leukocytes (lymphocytes, monocytes, macrophages, and granulocytes), and a cell type termed as metrial gland cells in some species, as well as stromal fibroblasts and blood vessels.[35] Although the decidual reaction begins most intensely at the implantation site, in all species exhibiting this reaction, decidualization eventually expands throughout the endometrium completely surrounding the conceptus and remains most marked in the placental bed. This latter component of the decidua, the decidua basalis, remains as the most important maternal counterpart of the fetomaternal interface.

Histological, endocrinological, and biochemical events associated with deciduogenesis during pregnancy or artificial induction of deciduoma during pseudopregnancy have been well documented and reviewed,[36-40] so also the life history of decidual cells.[41] It has been shown from 3HTdR labeling experiments that typical stromal type decidual cells (henceforth called decidual cells) are the end products of proliferation and differentiation of stromal fibroblast-like precursors within the progestational endometrium.[42-47] Whether these precursors represent a subset of or all endometrial stromal cells remains undetermined. It is pertinent to point out that an ultrastructural evidence of stromal cell transformation (predecidual stage) shortly after implantation is seen focally in the subepithelial (periluminal) stroma and occasionally surrounding the capillaries, rather than throughout the endometrial stroma, as illustrated in FIGURE 1.

Decidual cells are best identifiable from their distinctive ultrastructural features,[39,48,49] and using these features, we have reidentified these cells in serial 1 μm thick Epon sections at the light microscope level. Their morphology in semithin sections is very similar to that noted for many cells in smear or cytocentrifuge preparations of single cell suspensions of the decidua or deciduoma dissociated with a mild collagenase treatment indicating that these cells can indeed be recovered in the latter preparations. In both preparations they are recognizable as slightly vacuolated, occasionally binucleate cells of ovoid appearance. Their nuclei are eccentric in position, round or ovoid in shape, and have uniformly dispersed chromatin containing one or more nucleoli. In smears or cytocentrifuge preparations stained with Giemsa these cells show a basophilic cytoplasm, and their sizes range between 12-30 μm in diameter (80% of the cells ranging between 15-20 μm), with 5-6% of the cells being binucleate on d12 of gestation in the CBA mouse decidua basalis.[50] The morphology of these cells is illustrated in FIGURE 2. These cells are nonphagocytic, whereas macrophages within the decidua are all capable of phagocytosing latex particles. Although presenting a similar size range, macrophages are highly vacuolated cells with an abundant, lighter staining cytoplasm containing a convoluted or occasionally ovoid nucleus. Other leukocytes (lymphocytes, monocytes, and granulocytes) and occasionally encountered metrial gland cells (ovoid cells, 25-50 μm in diameter, containing numerous diastase-resistant, Periodic-Acid-Schiff positive granules in pale cytoplasm) are easily distinguishable from decidual cells in single cell preparations.

Our ability to identify decidual cells in single cell preparations provided us with a tool to ask the following question: What is the ultimate origin of decidual cell precursors? Are they descendants of stem cells residing in the uterus or migrating from an extrauterine source? In view of their possible immunological function to be described later on, we tested the hypothesis that the stem cells for the endometrial precursors of the decidual cells may originate from the bone marrow.[51] The H-2 phenotype of decidual cells was examined at the morphological level with a radioautographic immunolabeling technique applied to single cell suspensions of collagenase dispersed deciduoma induced in pseudopregnant radiation bone marrow chimeras 4 to 10 weeks after bone marrow reconstitution. Whole-body irradiation of parental strain mice followed by bone marrow reconstitution from F_1 strain donors was employed to produce chimerism. The extent of chimerism in decidual cells of individual mice, identifiable on the basis of donor H-2 phenotype went hand in hand with that noted for macrophages in the decidua as well as splenic lymphocytes, leading to the conclusion that precursors of decidual cells, at least those recovered from the collagenase-dispersed deciduoma, were ultimate descendants of the bone marrow under these experi-

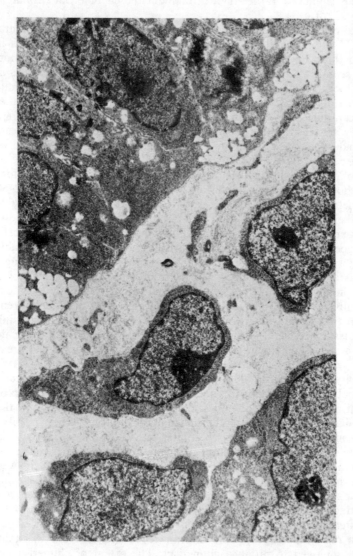

FIGURE 1A. Low power electron micrograph of the CBA mouse uterus on late day 4 of gestation showing stromal cell transformation (predecidual cells) in the periluminal stroma. Subepithelial stromal cells show nuclear enlargement and peripheral condensation of chromatin. They also begin to take a more rounded appearance than fibroblasts; × 6400.

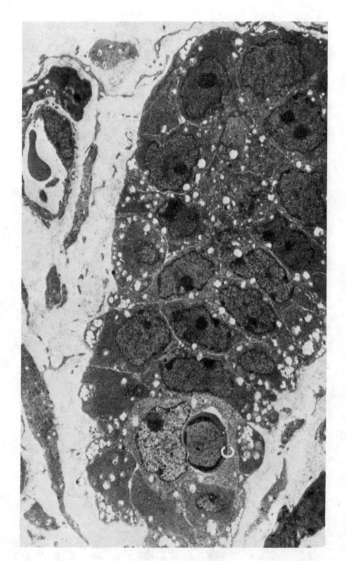

FIGURE 1B. Low power electron micrograph of the CBA mouse uterus on late day 4 of gestation showing a discrete focus of stromal cell transformation in the endometrium surrounding a capillary (C); × 3250.

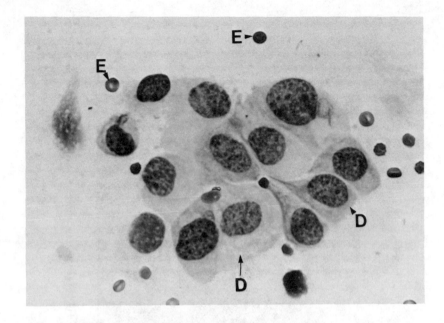

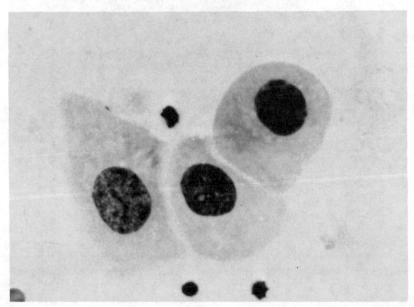

FIGURE 2. Murine decidual cells in a smear of collagenase-dispersed decidua at day 12 of gestation. Top: × 750; Bottom: × 1200. D = decidual cell; E = erythrocyte.

mental conditions. To reconcile this observation with the very slow turnover rate reported for endometrial stromal cells,[52] one may invoke two possibilities. (1) There may be a cyclic migration of these stem cells to the uterus throughout reproductive life. This remains a viable possibility, because stromal-cell turnover is known to be enhanced under the influence of ovarian hormones.[52,53] (2) Alternatively, the major migratory event may occur during ontogeny or early postnatal life, without excluding the possibility that a small amount of migration may also occur during reproductive life. In either case, a stem cell migration from the bone marrow to the endometrium in our experimental animals may have been amplified owing to a depletion of local precursors destroyed by irradiation of the uterus. We are currently testing these possibilities using prenatally or neonatally reconstituted mice and adult radiation chimeras made fertile with syngeneic ovary transplants.[c] Recently two laboratories have examined the extent of bone marrow contribution to the decidua of pregnancy or deciduoma of pseudopregnancy in bone marrow-reconstituted mice using allotypic markers for the cellular isoenzyme glucose phosphate isomerase (GPI)[54,55] or phosphoglycerate kinase (PGK)[55] examined on lysates of whole decidual tissue[54,55] or dissociated decidual cell suspensions obtained with mild collagenase treatment.[54] A successful pregnancy was attainable only in those animals that received H-2 antibody treatment[54] (rather than irradiation) or a low sublethal dose of irradiation[55] prior to reconstitution. Although the isoenzyme methods did not permit an examination of the phenotypic identity of the individual cells, they allowed an estimation of the overall extent of chimerism at the tissue level to reveal (1) that the degree of chimerism in the nondispersed decidua or deciduoma as well as in the fibrous decidual matrix remaining after collagenase dispersion of these tissues was small or negligible in animals that showed variable degrees of chimerism in splenic white cells or bone marrow cells; and (2) that variable but substantial bone marrow contribution was seen in the collagenase-dispersed decidua or deciduoma,[54] the degree of chimerism in most cases being comparable to that for splenic leukocytes, as had been documented in our studies at the single cell level.[51] These results indicate (1) that the bulk of the decidual stromal elements (fibroblasts, fibrocytes, and blood vessels left behind after collagenase dispersion) does not have a bone marrow genealogy, and (2) that collagenase dispersion preferentially isolates marrow-derived elements that may represent a minor subpopulation of cells within the decidua or the deciduoma. Evidently an *in situ* labeling of the individual cells of the decidua for the donor phenotype is needed to trace the temporal and geographic distribution as well as the morphological features of the marrow-derived cells within the decidua, other than those readily identifiable as leukocytes or metrial gland cells. The latter cell class has also been shown to have a bone marrow genealogy on the basis of a donor-related morphological marker in chimeric mice reconstituted with rat marrow.[56] In our experience, the incidence of metrial gland cells is extremely low in the collagenase-dispersed mouse decidua or deciduoma.

[c] *Note added in proof:* Results of these experiments reveal that at least a subset of decidual cells of pregnancy are descendants of stem cells in the fetal liver or the bone marrow, which migrate to the uterus during prenatal and postnatal lives.

SURFACE MARKER CHARACTERISTICS OF DECIDUAL CELLS: MARKERS SHARED WITH LYMPHOMYELOID CELLS AND UNIQUE TO DECIDUAL CELLS

In view of the bone marrow genealogy of the decidual cells recovered by collagenase dispersion, as well as their immunosuppressor function to be described later, we explored the familial relationship of these cells to other cells of the immune system by examining a battery of cell-surface markers recognized on lymphomyeloid cells:[50] Thy-1 (present on thymocytes and epidermal dendritic cells—a stromal cell class in the epidermis derived from the bone marrow), Mac-1 (expressed on macrophages and granulocytes), Lyt-1 and Lyt-2 (present on T-lymphocyte subsets), I-A (present on B lymphocytes and marrow-derived, antigen-presenting accessory cells of the immune system, e.g. certain macrophages, epidermal Langerhans' cells, dendritic reticular cells, and follicular dendritic cells), and I-J antigens (expressed on certain populations of suppressor T lymphocytes). Dispersed cell populations of the CBA mouse decidua at 8-14 days of syngeneic pregnancy were either labeled directly by exposure to ^{125}I-labeled monoclonal antibodies against Thy-1, Mac-1, or Lyt antigens or indirectly by a sequential exposure to monoclonal anti I-A^k (Ia.17) or monospecific anti I-J^k antibodies and ^{125}I-labeled protein A. The presence and the density of these markers were examined at the morphological level in radioautographic preparations. Decidual cells were found to be Thy-1$^\pm$ (13-73% positive, the incidence rising with advancing gestation in the decidua basalis), Mac-1$^\pm$ (present on 6-11% on day 8 and 17-32% on day 12), I-A$^-$, I-J$^-$, and Lyt$^-$. Macrophages within the decidua were Thy-1$^-$, Lyt$^-$, Mac-1$^+$, and I-A$^\pm$ (present on 5-61% of cells, the incidence rising with advancing gestation). These surface properties of decidual cells along with the presence of F$_c$ receptors, and absence of C$_3$ receptors, and the presence of a unique marker, Dec-1, to be described below, distinguish them from most other stromal-type immunoregulatory cells such as Langerhans' cells (I-A$^+$, FcR$^+$, C$_3$R$^+$, Mac-1$^-$, Thy-1$^-$), follicular dendritic cells (I-A$^+$, FcR$^+$, Thy-1$^-$, Mac-1$^-$, Dec-1$^-$), and dendritic reticular cells (I-A$^+$, FcR$^-$, C$_3$R$^-$, Thy-1$^-$, Lyt$^-$, Mac-1$^-$). A substantial subpopulation of decidual cells, however, share a few properties (I-A$^-$, Thy-1$^+$) with another marrow-derived stromal type cell in the epidermis described as epidermal dendritic cells, which remain to be investigated for other surface markers such as Mac-1, Dec-1, and FcR. Thy-1 positivity may also be related to the fibroblastic genealogy of decidual cells,[57] because certain embryonic fibroblasts in culture are also known to express this marker.

To explore whether decidual cells express lineage-specific differentiation marker(s), we resorted to the hybridoma technology.[58,59] Virgin CBA mice were immunized against syngeneic decidual cells with the hope that having undergone no decidual cell reaction, they might respond to the immunization protocol with a low probability of producing irrelevant antibodies. Two monoclonal antibodies of the IgG-2b isotype secreted by clones 16F12 and 2G4F8 were examined for their binding characteristics and the tissue distribution of binding after a sandwich labeling with FITC-protein A on frozen sections followed by fluorescence microscopy[58] or with ^{125}I-protein A on single cell suspensions followed by radioautography.[59] At the tissue level, both antibodies showed specific and moderately strong focal binding to decidual cell groups clustering around blood vessels on the lateral edge of the decidua basalis and weaker binding to cells of the decidua capsularis at day 8 of gestation in the CBA mouse. Stronger labeling of the decidua basalis was noted on day 14, but the pattern was somewhat different with the two antibodies. This was seen as circumscribed bands with 16F12 and on scattered cells with 2G4F8. Trophoblast cells of the placenta were labeled with neither antibody.

An examination of radioautographic binding to single cell suspensions of the placenta, decidua, and lymphomyeloid organs revealed that both antibodies recognized antigen(s) unique to the decidual cell lineage in numerous species—mice, humans, and rats. The incidence of antigen-bearing decidual cells increased with gestational age in CBA, C_3H, and CD_1 mice between day 8 (25-29% for 16F12 and 0-20% for 2G4F8) and day 14 (63-70% for 16F12, and 18-65% for 2G4F8) and in humans between 6 wk (24-26% for 16F12 and 19-24% for 2G4F8) and 12.5 wk (58% with 16F12 and 18% with 2G4F8), but some decline was noted in Sprague Dawley or Lewis rats between day 8 (32-69% for both antibodies) and day 14 (27-48% for 16F12 and 12-13% for 2G4F8). There was no significant labeling of trophoblast cells of the placenta or leukocytes within the decidua in any of these species. Little or no labeling of any cell type was seen on lymphomyeloid cells of the virgin or pregnant CBA mice, but a consistent labeling of a rare blast-type cell in the blood was observed with both these antibodies, raising the speculation that this cell may represent the circulating precursor for the marrow-derived lineage of decidual cells or all marrow-derived stromal type immunoregulatory cells.[59] In this context it is pertinent to mention that a decidual cell reaction has occasionally been noted at extrauterine sites, for example, on the broad ligament or the ovarian surface during normal human pregnancy, during ectopic tubal pregnancy,[60] and also in the placental bed of primary abdominal pregnancy.[61]

It remains to be determined whether antibodies 16F12 and 2G4F8 are recognizing the same or different antigens on the decidual cell surface. 16F12-defined antigenic marker has been termed as Dec-1.[59] A conservation of these antigen(s) during speciation may indicate their functional importance. This possibility as well as the molecular nature of the antigen(s) remain to be explored. Because the Dec-1$^+$ decidual cells are initially seen to appear as foci around blood vessels,[58] it will be of interest to examine with double labeling techniques whether this marker is identifying the marrow-derived decidual cell lineage *in situ.*

KINETICS OF ACCUMULATION OF DECIDUAL CELLS AND VARIOUS LEUKOCYTE SUBSETS IN THE MURINE DECIDUA DURING SYNGENEIC AND ALLOGENEIC PREGNANCY

In spite of reported histological differences in the leukocyte accumulation in the homozygous versus heterozygous placenta,[62] their migration potential into the decidua remains undetermined. Studies on the human decidual leu-kocyte surface markers *in situ*[63,64] have provided valuable qualitative infor-mation; however, the relative contribution of the various cell populations and their subsets to the decidual development in any species remains unknown. This information is particularly important for the decidua basalis, which forms the bed for the placental trophoblast. As a basis for further functional studies, we evaluated the contribution of decidual cells and numerous leu-kocyte subsets (characterized on the basis of cell-surface markers) to the development of murine decidua during syngeneic (CBA♀ × CBA♂) and allogeneic (CBA ♀ × C57BL/6 ♂) pregnancy.[65] Collagenase-dispersed de-cidua were subjected to total and differential counts and cell-surface labeling for a radioautographic identification of various markers: surface-IgM on B lymphocytes, Thy-1 on T lymphocytes, neither marker on null lymphocytes, Lyt- (1 or 2, or 1,2) antigens on T-cell subsets, and Mac-1 and I-A on macrophages, using ^{125}I-labeled monoclonal antibodies or a sandwich labeling with [^{125}I]protein A. The total cellularity of the decidua basalis showed a biphasic rise in both pregnancies, with peaks on day 11 and day 15-16, but the allopregnant decidua showed a higher accumulation of all cell types, indicating that an allogeneic conceptus causes an augmented deciduogenesis. The number of decidual cells, the most frequent cell class, rose to a peak on day 11 followed by a decline possibly due to cell death. The number of lymphocytes, the next frequent cell class, showed a parallel pattern initially, followed by a sharp secondary rise on day 16. This rise may be due to a withdrawal of progesterone, an antiinflammatory hormone. Null cells pre-dominated among decidual lymphocytes (45-80%), as well as in the proges-tational endometrium (53%), indicating a hormonal control of their accumulation. The frequencies of B cells (10-13%) were low, and T cells (25-45%) were comparable to that in the blood, with Lyt-1$^+$,2$^-$ class being the most common T-cell subset. Allopregnant decidua also showed a late rise in the total number of Lyt-2$^+$, 1$^-$ cells, which may have a suppressor function. Macrophages, the next common leukocyte class, all expressed Mac-1. There number rose to a plateau by day 12, but at a higher level in allopregnancy. I-A (needed for antigen presentation) was expressed by an increasing pro-portion (5-60%) of macrophages with advancing gestation.

FIGURE 3 illustrates radioautographs of various cell types within the decidua labeled for numerous cell-surface markers.

IMMUNOLOGICAL FUNCTION OF THE MAJOR LEUKOCYTE SUBSETS IN THE DECIDUA

"Null" Lymphocytes

As mentioned earlier, this subset represents the most predominant class of lymphoid cells in the progestational endometrium as well as the decidua

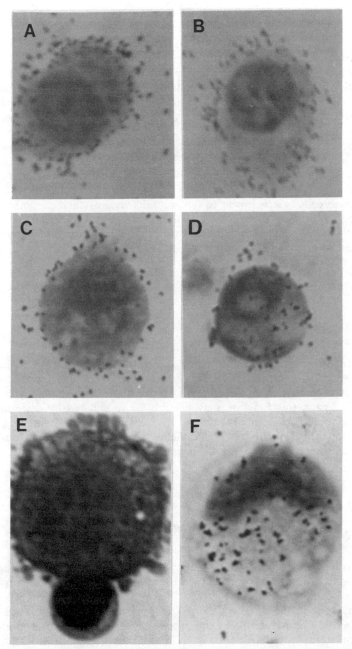

FIGURE 3. Radioautographic preparations of cells of the decidua labeled for various cell surface markers ($\times$ 1500). **A-C:** Dec-1$^+$ decidual cells; **A:** from CBA mouse; **B:** from Lewis rat; and **C** from human. **D:** Thy-1$^+$ CBA mouse decidual cell. **E:** An NK lineage cell (S-IgM$^-$, Thy-1$^-$, or null lymphocyte binding to a YAC-1 lymphoma target) from the CBA mouse decidua. **F:** I-A$^+$ macrophage in the CBA mouse decidua.

throughout the course of murine gestation. At least two important functional subpopulations have now been identified within this subset. One class, exhibiting a granular morphology and bearing F_c receptors is found to exert a local immunosuppressor function against the generation of cytotoxic T cells in an MHC unrestricted manner, apparently requiring a trophoblast-decidual interaction for its appearance in the endometrium.[66,67] The suppressor function seems to be mediated by a 100 kDa factor capable of blocking the lymphocyte response to interleukin-2 (IL-2),[68] a growth factor recognized to be required for lymphocyte activation and proliferation before the generation of cytotoxic cells. A second functional class of null lymphocytes within the decidua belongs to the natural killer (NK) lineage cells. We have observed that this cell lineage appears in the decidua in large numbers.[23] Although target structures recognized by NK cells are expressed by midgestational murine trophoblast,[20] trophoblast cells *in situ* appear to remain unharmed by their presence within the decidua, because their activation is prevented by suppressor factors released by the decidual cells and macrophages.[23] These factors have now been identified as prostaglandins, primarily PGE_2, as discussed later.

Lyt-1⁺ Subset of T Lymphocytes

As mentioned earlier, the major subset of T lymphocytes within the decidua are Lyt-1⁺,2⁻ cells. These cells may perform one or more functions that remain to be investigated. The first is production of growth factors such as IL-2. Again, this function may possibly be modulated by decidual cell-derived suppressor molecules such as PGE_2. The second is induction of T-suppressor cells[69] (of the Lyt-2⁺,1⁻ phenotype), which are found to increase in the late gestational decidua of allogeneic pregnancy.

Macrophages

Two functional macrophage subpopulations have now been identified in the decidua, although it is not clear whether they may represent two functional stages of the same cells: (1) an I-A⁺ class,[65] thus capable of processing antigens,[70] the incidence of which rises with advancing gestation, (these cells may play an important role in the processing of fetal antigens expressed at the fetomaternal interface), and (2) an immunosuppressor class, which along with decidual cells, can suppress the activation of lymphocytes[23,71,72] and the subsequence generation of functional killer cells. The suppressor factors, at least in part, have been identified as prostaglandins,[23,72] as elaborated later.

IMMUNOREGULATORY FUNCTION OF DECIDUAL CELLS

An immunoprotective function of the decidua for the fetoplacental survival was proposed many years ago;[3,30] attempts, however, to dissect the role of the various cellular constituents as well as the precise mechanisms involved have only begun recently. Crude extracts of decidual tissue have been shown to suppress the antibody response of B lymphocytes to the antigen dinitrophenol-polylysine,[73] proliferative response of T lymphocytes to allogeneic cells in mixed lymphocyte reaction (MLR), or to polyclonal T-cell mitogens.[74] Similarly, culture supernatants of murine decidual cells have been shown to suppress the MLR in an MHC-nonspecific manner[75-77] without any effect on the killer function of cytotoxic T cells.[75] The suppressor activity has been partially identified in the 40-50 kDa as well 300^+ kDa fractions of the supernatant.[77] Recently we have initiated a series of studies employing enriched or highly purified cell populations of the decidua to explore the nature of the immunosuppression, the identity of the suppressor cells, and the suppressor molecules as well as their mode of action.[2,23,29,35,72] These studies, to be summarized below, indicate that decidual cells may exercise a crucial immunoprotective function *in situ.*

Decidual Cells Suppress Lymphocyte Alloreactivity *In Vitro*

We have shown that 85-90% pure midgestational mouse decidual cells fractionated by Ficoll-paque or discontinuous percoll density gradient centrifugation and inactivated with mitomycin C or gamma irradiation are capable of abrogating the MLR (proliferation of lymphocytes in mixed lymphocyte cultures) in a genetically unrestricted and dose-dependent manner.[2] This effect is reproducible with (48-72 hr) culture supernatants of decidual cells (V. Colavincenzo and P. K. Lala, unpublished data). These findings have been followed up in more detail employing human decidual cell populations with a higher degree (92-97%) of purity.[29,72] Normal decidual tissue recovered from therapeutic abortion materials at 4.5-12 weeks of gestation and dispersed with 0.3% collagenase, when fractionated on a column of Ficoll-paque, had a high natural incidence of decidual cells during early gestation (*e.g.* 88-94% at 4.5-7.5 wks). This incidence then declined sharply (to 45-55% at 8-8.5 wks and 20-25% at 9.5-12 wks), primarily due to an increasing contamination of macrophages and granulocytes, which could be removed by plastic adherence. The plastic adherent fractions, however, still retained a high proportion of decidual cells. Ficoll-paque separated decidual cells, or in some experiments, their plastic-nonadherent or plastic-adherent fractions were inactivated with 2800 rads γ-rays. These cells were added in various doses (10^3-10^5 cells) to mixed lymphocyte cultures (MLC) set up by mixing HLA disparate human peripheral blood lymphocytes at various ratios of responder (R) and 2800 Rγ-irradiated stimulator (S) cells as follows: 10^5R + 10^5S; 10^5R + 1.5 × 10^5S; 2 × 10^5R + 1.5 × 10^5S. Sources of decidual cells (D), R or S were completely unrelated. Addition of decidual cells or their fractions led to a dose-dependent suppression of the MLR ([^{3}H]TdR uptake given by β counts) in all experiments measured on days 3, 4, or 5, a stronger suppression being noted with purer decidual cell preparations. Results of one experiment (day 4 MLR) are illustrated in FIGURE 4. These results suggested that the decidual cells, and most likely also the macrophages within the decidua were capable of suppressing lymphocyte alloreactivity in a dose-dependent and MHC-unrestricted manner.

MLR Suppression by Decidual Cells Is Mediated by Prostaglandins, Primarily PGE₂

A series of experiments was undertaken to identify the nature of the suppressor molecules. (1) Indomethacin (10^{-5}M concentration), an inhibitor

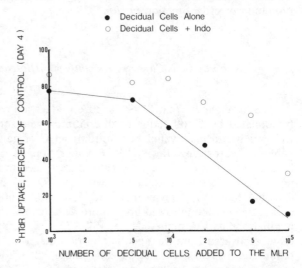

FIGURE 4. MLR (CPM, [^{3}H]TdR uptake on day 4 MLC set up mixing 10^5 stimulator 1.5 × 10^5 responder lymphocytes) in the presence of increasing doses of human decidual cells of six-week gestational age ± indomethacin (10^{-5}M).

of prostaglandin synthesis, when added to the MLC, relieved the decidual cell-mediated suppression to a major extent (FIG. 4) or completely in some experiments (TABLE 1), although by itself it had no direct effect on the MLR. (2) A similar restoration of the MLR was also achieved in the presence of an anti-PGE₂ antibody at different dilutions (kindly provided by Dr. T. G. Kennedy), indicating that most or all of the suppression was accountable by the production of PGE₂ (TABLE 1). (3) PGE₂ concentration measurable in these cultures on day 4 (with kind collaboration of Dr. T. G. Kennedy using a radioimmune assay) went hand in hand with the degree of suppression,

TABLE 1. Reversal of Decidual Cell-Mediated Suppression of MLR in the Presence of Indomethacin (10^{-5}M) or α-PGE$_2$ Antibody

Added number of decidual cells (8.5 wk gestation)	MLR (Percent of Control)				
	R + S	R + S + NRS	R + S + α-PGE$_2$	R + S + Indo	
0	100.	—	—	103	
6 × 10^3	77.0	78.4[a]	87.3[a]	—	
12 × 10^3	67.2	70.0[b]	98.2[b]	—	
25 × 10^3	44.8	51.6[c]	94.8[c]	98.0	

[a] 1:1200 dilution
[b] 1:12 dilution
[c] Undiluted concentrations of NRS (normal rabbit serum) or α-PGE$_2$ Ab raised in rabbits; Indo = indomethacin (10^{-5}M).

TABLE 2. Decidual Cell-Mediated MLR Suppression versus the Level of PGE_2 Measurable in the MLC

| Experiment number | Decidual cells | | 4-day MLR (CPM) | | R + S + D, as percent of control | PGE_2 concentration in the culture[a] (ng/ml) |
	Gestation age (weeks)	Number added	R + S alone	R + S + D		
1	7.5	25×10^3	31,773	8,431	26.5	27.1
2	8.5	50×10^3	51,765	7,011	13.7	37.6
3	8.5	50×10^3	49,271	9,851	19.7	28.0
4	10.0	50×10^3	34,327	9,235	26.9	30.0

[a] The PGE_2 concentration in the cultures in the absence of decidual cells was negligible in these experiments (a mean of 0.28 ng/ml in R + S alone and 0.18 ng/ml in the tissue culture medium containing 10% human serum).

only minute levels of PGE_2 being detectable in control cultures in the absence of suppressor cells (TABLE 2). Furthermore, the PGE_2 concentration on day 4, generated by a fixed number of decidual cells from an individual tissue sample, was identical when cultured alone or cultured in the MLC (data not shown), indicating that cells in the MLC did not influence the PGE_2 production by decidual cells. (4) Most likely, the PGE_2 level detected on day 4 reflected a balance between production and degradation, because a higher concentration of chemically pure PGE_2 was needed at the beginning of the MLC to achieve a similar degree of suppression (TABLE 3). This suppression, again, was dose dependent.

TABLE 3. MLR Suppression in the Presence of PGE_2

Dose of PGE_2 added (ng/ml culture)	4-day MLR (CPM $\times$ 10^{-3})	MLR as percent of control
0	19.2	100
75	18.0	94
150	13.2	69
300	10.4	55
750	6.0	32
1500	5.4	29
3000	2.7	14

PGE_2-Mediated MLR Suppression by Decidual Cells Prevents the Generation of Cytotoxic T Lymphocytes in the MLC

The presence of cytotoxic T cells is demonstrable in the day 7 MLC, using ^{51}Cr-labeled Con A-stimulated lymphoblasts (of the stimulator phenotype) as targets in a ^{51}Cr release assay (conventionally referred to as the cell-mediated lysis or CML). This phenomenon is believed to represent the final effector phase of the allograft rejection response *in vivo*. TABLE 4 presents the results of one experiment showing a suppression of the CML in the presence of decidual cells or their fractions, reversible in the presence of indomethacin. A higher suppression was noted in the presence of the nonadherent than of the adherent fraction.

Decidual Cells and Decidual Macrophages Suppress the Functional Activation of Natural Killer Lymphocytes by a Prostaglandin-Mediated Mechanism

We examined whether NK lineage lymphocytes appear within the murine decidua, and if so, what prevents them from expressing their killer function *in situ.*[23] NK lineage lymphocytes (null lymphocytes capable of forming conjugates with YAC-1 lymphoma targets) were identified with a radioautographic method that labeled B and T lymphocytes leaving the null lymphocytes unlabeled[20] (illustrated in FIG. 3). The incidence of NK lineage cells was found to be as high among the nucleated cells of the murine midgestational decidua as in the normal spleen. Their killer function, however, (measured with a ^{51}Cr release assay using ^{51}Cr-labeled YAC-1 lymphoma targets) was found to have declined to low levels in the decidua at days 10-14 of gestation. The reason for this inactivation was found to be due to the presence of NK suppressor cells in the decidua. Ficoll-paque-separated decidual cells from the CBA or CD$_1$ mouse or their plastic adherent or nonadherent fraction, when mixed with normal splenic effector cells of either

TABLE 4. Effects of the Presence of Cells of the Decidua or Their Fractions ± Indomethacin (10^{-5}M) in the MLC on the Generation of CML^a

MLC set up	CML (percent of control) exhibited by cells of 7-day MLC
R + S	100
R + S + Indo	109
R + S + D	23
R + S + D + Indo	105
R + S + D$_1$	40
R + S + D$_1$ + Indo	137
R + S + D$_2$	62
R + S + D$_2$ + Indo	98

^{a} R = 1.5×10^5 responder cells; S = 10^5 irradiated stimulator cells; D = 5×10^4 irradiated unfractionated decidual cells (6.5 week gestational age); D$_1$ = plastic nonadherent fraction (97% decidual cells, 3% lymphocytes); D$_2$ = plastic adherent fraction (62% decidual cells, 25% macrophages, 11% granulocytes, and 2% lymphocytes).

mouse strain (at 1:1 ratio) led to a suppression of the NK activity tested immediately after mixing or after a 20-hour coculture. This suppression was completely reversible in the presence of indomethacin (10^{-5}M) indicating its mediation by prostaglandins released by decidual cells as well as decidual macrophages. Similar to the experiments described for the human decidua, there was an excellent correlation of this suppression with the PGE$_2$ concentration measurable in the overnight cultures of murine decidual cells. Again, this suppression was effective across strain barriers irrespective of the MHC phenotype of the effector cells.

Because PGE$_2$ appears to inhibit an activation of both alloreactive and natural killer lymphocytes, this inhibition is possibly exerted by common mechanism(s). These may include (1) suppression of the development IL-2 receptors on lymphocytes of both these lineages, the activation of which is IL-2 dependent, (2) inhibition of production of IL-2 by IL-2-secreting T cells,[78] and (3) blocking the response of IL-2 receptor-bearing lymphocytes to IL-2.[79] We have currently obtained evidence in support of the first and second, but against the third mechanism (R. S. Parhar, T. G. Kennedy, and P. K. Lala, submitted for publication).

IN VIVO SIGNIFICANCE OF THE PGE$_2$-MEDIATED IMMUNOSUPPRESSION BY DECIDUAL CELLS

It has recently been shown that PGE$_2$ and progesterone can act synergistically in suppressing lymphocyte activation *in vitro.*[80] It is highly likely that a local immunosuppression by the products of the decidua (most importantly PGE$_2$) as well as the trophoblast (progesterone) may jointly prevent an activation of maternal lymphocytes with cytotoxic potentials *in situ.* To test whether the PGE$_2$-mediated suppression has an *in vivo* relevance, we examined the outcome of continuous administration of indomethacin in the drinking water at various doses on the course of pregnancy in random bred CD$_1$ female mice (J. Scodras and P. K. Lala, unpublished data). A nontoxic regimen (14 μg/ml of water) starting in the morning of day 5 after the appearance of the vaginal plug (*i.e.* approximately one day after implantation) was found to result in abortions in 70-75% of the mice, followed by a partial or a complete resorption of the embryos by day 8. Cells isolated from the endometrium of these mice on day 8 exhibited very high levels of natural killer activity, reminiscent of lymphokine-activated killer cells, which can kill a variety of tumor cells and embryonic cells. These results, although not providing a cause and effect relationship, are highly suggestive of the local PGE$_2$-mediated immunoprotective role of the decidua for the fetoplacental unit. We have reported a very similar mechanism exerted by host-derived macrophages in protecting the tumor from the host immune apparatus.[81,82,83]

EPILOGUE

Most or all cellular constituents of the decidua appear to play a local immunoregulatory role for the survival of the conceptus. Decidual cells, the unique cells of the pregnant endometrium that have evolved by necessity, are multifunctional cells serving nutritive, endocrine, and immune functions for the sustenance of pregnancy. Further studies of decidual cells at the cellular and molecular levels using a multidisciplinary approach should be rewarding. At the cellular level, tracing the complete genealogy of decidual cells *in vivo* as well as during artificial decidualization *in vitro,* and at the molecular level, the molecular nature of decidual cell-specific differentiation marker(s) as well as the genes coding for the marker(s) remain as fruitful areas of investigation.

REFERENCES

1. WOODRUFF, M. F. A. 1958. Proc. R. Soc. London (Biol.) **148:** 68-75.
2. LALA, P. K., S. CHATTERJEE-HASROUNI, M. KEARNS, B. MONTGOMERY & V. COLA-VINCENZO. 1983. Immunol. Rev. **75:** 87-116.
3. BEER, A. E. & R. E. BILLINGHAM. 1976. Prentice-Hall Inc. Englewood Cliffs.
4. Immunol. Rev. 1983. Vol. 75.
5. WEGMANN, T. G. & T. J. GILL, Eds. 1983. Reproductive Immunology. Oxford University Press. Oxford, England.
6. Contr. Gynec. Obstet. 1985. Vol. 14.
7. GILL, T. J. & T. G. WEGMANN, Eds. 1986. Immunoregulation and Fetal Survival. Oxford University Press. Oxford, England. In press.
8. LALA, P. K., M. KEARNS & V. COLAVINCENZO. 1984. Am. J. Anat. **170:** 501-517.
9. BEER, A. E. & R. E. BILLINGHAM. 1974. J. Reprod. Fertil. Suppl. **21:** 59-88.
10. HEYNER, S. 1980. In Immunological Aspects of Infertility and Fertility Regulation. D. S. Dhinsda & G. F. B. Schumacher, Eds.: 183-203. Elsevier/North-Holland. Amsterdam.
11. CHATTERJEE-HASROUNI, S. & P. K. LALA. 1979. J. Exp. Med. **149:** 1238-1253.
12. CHATTERJEE-HASROUNI, S. & P. K. LALA. 1981. J. Immunol. **127:** 2070-2073.
13. CHATTERJEE-HASROUNI, S. & P. K. LALA. 1982. J. Exp. Med. **155:** 1679-1689.
14. COLAVINCENZO, V. & P. K. LALA. 1984. Anat. Rec. **108**(3): 33A.
15. COLAVINCENZO, V. & P. K. LALA. 1985. Anat. Rec. **211**(3): 42A-43A.
16. SUNDERLAND, C. A., W. G. REDMAN & G. M. STIRRAT. 1981. J. Immunol. **127:** 2614-2615.
17. MONTGOMERY, B. & P. K. LALA. 1983. J. Immunol. **131:** 2348-2355.
18. FAULK, W. P. & J. A. McINTYRE. 1983. Immunol. Rev. **75:** 139-175.
19. BULMER, J. N. & P. M. JOHNSON. 1985. Placenta **6:** 127-140.
20. CHATTERJEE-HASROUNI, S., R. PARHAR & P. K. LALA. 1984. Cell Immunol. **84:** 264-275.
21. STITES, D. P. & P. K. SIITERI. 1983. Immunol. Rev. **75:** 117-138.
22. CHAOUAT, G. & J. P. KOLB. 1985. J. Immunol. **135:** 215-222.
23. SCODRAS, J. M., R. S. PARHAR & P. K. LALA. 1985. Anat. Rec. **211**(3): 171A-172A.
24. GAMBEL, P., B. A. CROY, W. D. MOORE, R. D. HUNZIKER, T. G. WEGMANN & J. ROSSANT. 1985. Cell Immunol. **93:** 303-314.
25. LOEB, L. 1907. Zentralbl. Allg. Pathol. Pathol. Anat. **18:** 563.
26. KRAICER, P. F. & M. C. SHELESNYAK. 1958. J. Endocrinol. **17:** 324.
27. FINN, C. A. & D. G. PORTER. 1975. The Uterus. 74-95. Elek Science. London.
28. KING, B. F. 1982. Bibl. Anat. **22:** 13-28.
29. LALA, P. K., M. KEARNS & R. S. PARHAR. 1986. In Immunoregulation and Fetal Survival. T. J. Gill and T. G. Wegmann, Eds. Oxford University Press. Oxford, England. In press.
30. KIRBY, D. R. S., W. D. BILLINGTON & D. A. JAMES. 1966. Transplantation **4:** 713-718.
31. BEER, A. E. & J. O. SIO. 1982. Biol. Reprod. **26:** 15-27.
32. FINN, C. A. 1980. Prog. Reprod. Biol. **7:** 253-261.
33. PIJENBORG, R., W. B. ROBERTSON & I. BROSENS. 1985. Placenta **6:** 155-162.
34. KIRBY, D. R. S. & T. P. COWELL. 1968. In Epithelial-Mesenchymal Interactions. R. Fleischmajer, and R. E. Billingham, Eds.: 64-77. Williams and Wilkins. Baltimore.
35. LALA, P. K. & M. KEARNS. 1985. Contr. Gynec. Obstet. **14:** 1-15.
36. KREHBIEL, R. H. 1937. Physiol. Zool. **5:** 212-235.
37. DEFEO, V. J. 1967. In Cellular Biology of the Uterus. R. M. Wynn, Ed.: 191-290. Meredith Publishing Co. New York.
38. FINN, C. A. 1971. Adv. Reprod. Biol. **5:** 1-26.
39. O'SHEA, J. D., R. G. KLEINFELD & H. A. MORROW. 1983. Am. J. Anat. **166:** 271-298.
40. BELL, S. C. 1983. Oxford Rev. Reprod. Bio. **5:** 220-271.
41. KEARNS, M. & P. K. LALA. 1983. Am. J. Reprod. Immunol. **3:** 78-82.
42. ZHINKIN, L. N. & N. A. SAMOSHKINA. 1967. J. Embryol. Exp. Morphol. **17:** 593-605.
43. GALASSI, L. 1968. Dev. Biol. **17:** 75-84.
44. SHELESNYAK, M. C., G. J. MARCUS & H. R. LINDER. 1970. In Ovo-Implantation. Human Gonadotropins and Prolactin. 118-129. Karger. Basel, Switzerland.
45. LEROY, F., C. BOGAERT, J. VANHOECK & C. DELCROIX. 1974. J. Reprod. Fertil. **38:** 441-449.

46. BULMER, D. & S. PEEL. 1974. J. Anat. **117:** 433-441.
47. DAS, R. M. & L. MARTIN. 1978. J. Reprod. Fertil. **53:** 125-128.
48. ENDERS, A. C. & S. SCHLAFKE. 1967. Am. J. Anat. **120:** 185-226.
49. JOLLIE, W. P. & S. A. BENCOSME. 1965. Am. J. Anat. **116:** 217-235.
50. KEARNS, M. & P. K. LALA. 1985. Am. J. Reprod. Immunol. Microbiol. **9:** 39-47.
51. KEARNS, M. & P. K. LALA. 1982. J. Exp. Med. **155:** 1537-1554.
52. DAS, R. M. 1972. J. Endocrinol. **55:** 21-30.
53. MARTIN, L., C. A. FINN & G. TRINDER. 1973. J. Endocrinol. **56:** 303-307.
54. GAMBEL, P., J. ROSSANT, R. D. HUNZIKER & T. G. WEGMANN. 1985. Transplantation **39:** 443-444.
55. FOWLIS, D. J. & J. D. ANSELL. 1985. Transplantation **39:** 445-446.
56. PEEL, S., I. J. STEWART & D. BULMER. 1983. Cell Tissue Res. **233:** 647.
57. BERNARD, O., M. SCHEID, M. A. RIPOCHE & D. BENNETT. 1978. J. Exp. Med. **148:** 580-591.
58. KEARNS, M. & P. K. LALA. 1985. Transplant. Proc. **17**(1): 911-915.
59. KEARNS, M., R. S. PARHAR & P. K. LALA. 1985. J. Immunol. **135:** 1046-1052.
60. AREY, L. B. 1965. Developmental Anatomy. 7th ed.: 129. W. B. Saunders Co. Philadelphia.
61. LIN, Y. Y., Y. C. CHU & W. Y. WANG. 1956. Chin. Med. J. **74:** 247-257.
62. KRCEK, J. P., A. D. DIXON & F. G. BIDDLE. 1983. J. Anat. **136:** 283-292.
63. BULMER, J. N. & C. A. SUNDERLAND. 1983. J. Reprod. Immunol. **5:** 383-387.
64. BULMER, J. N. & C. A. SUNDERLAND. 1984. Immunology **52:** 349-356.
65. KEARNS, M. & P. K. LALA. 1985. J. Reprod. Immunol. **8:** 213-234.
66. SLAPSYS, R. M. & D. A. CLARK. 1983. Am. J. Reprod. Immunol. **3:** 65-71.
67. CLARK, D. A., R. M. SLAPSYS, B. A. CROY, J. KRCEK & J. ROSSANT. 1984. Am. J. Reprod. Immunol. **5:** 78.
68. CLARK, D. A., A. CHAPUT, C. WALKER & K. L. ROSENTHAL. 1985. J. Immunol. **134:** 1659-1664.
69. EARDLEY, D. D., J. HUGENBERGER, L. MCVAY-BOUDREAU, F. W. SHEN, R. K. GERSHON & H. CANTOR. 1978. J. Exp. Med. **147:** 1106-1115.
70. ELCOCK, J. M. & R. F. SEARLE. 1985. Am. J. Reprod. Immunol. Microbiol. **7:** 99-103.
71. HUNT, J. S., L. S. MANNING & G. W. WOOD. 1984. Cell Immunol. **85:** 499-510.
72. PARHAR, R. S. & P. K. LALA. 1985. Anat. Rec. **211**(3): 147A.
73. GLOBERSON, A., S. ABAUMINGER, L. ABEL & S. PELEG. 1976. Eur. J. Immunol. **6:** 120-122.
74. GOLANDER, A., V. ZAKUTH, Y. SCHECHTER & Z. SPIRER. 1981. Eur. J. Immunol. **11:** 849-851.
75. KIRKWOOD, K. J. & S. C. BELL. 1981. J. Reprod. Immunol. **3:** 243-252.
76. BADET, M. T., S. C. BELL & W. D. BILLINGTON. 1983. J. Reprod. Fertil. **68:** 351-358.
77. BADET, M. T., S. C. BELL & W. D. BILLINGTON. 1983. Ann. Immunol. Inst. Pasteur (Paris) **134C**(3): 321-329.
78. MAKOUL, G. T., D. R. ROBINSON, A. K. BHALLA & L. H. GLIMCHER. 1985. J. Immunol. **134:** 2645-1650.
79. BRAUN, D. P. & J. E. HARRIS. 1984. J. Biol. Response Mod. **3**(5): 533-540.
80. FUJISAKI, S., K. KAWANO, Y. HARUYAMA & N. MORI. 1985. J. Reprod. Immunol. **7:** 15-26.
81. LALA, P. K., V. SANTER, H. LIBENSON & R. S. PARHAR. 1985. Cell Immunol. **93:** 250-264.
82. PARHAR, R. S. & P. K. LALA. 1985. Cell Immunol. **93:** 265-279.
83. LALA, P. K., R. S. PARHAR & P. SINGH. 1986. Cell Immunol. **99:** 108-118.

Concluding Remarks

G. J. MARCUS

Animal Research Centre
Agriculture Canada
Ottawa, Ontario, Canada K1A 0C6

At the beginning of this symposium, Dr. Shelesnyak retraced for us the avenues he followed over the years, revealing how much we owe to the maps of those explorations that he provided. Having been privileged to participate in constructing some of those maps, I am grateful for the opportunity to comment on the presentations today and to end with a reformulation or updating of the last model Shelesnyak showed, which dates from 1970.[1]

First of all, I thank the speakers for making my task of summarizing easier by providing me (in most cases) with information in advance and by giving lucid presentations. The diversity of the work presented, directed at so restricted a target as nidation, which is usually allotted only a small segment of the program at meetings on reproduction (when considered at all), encompasses a microcosm of biological research, in which virtually every discipline is brought to bear. This is clear from the different levels of approach seen today, viewing nidation from the macroperspective of the endocrine level and zeroing down to the microperspective of the molecular and microanatomic levels.

The first level is, of course, the most general and considers the temporal and hormonal aspects of nidation. Dr. Psychoyos' description of uterine receptivity and definition of markers or criteria thereof drew our attention to what has been, for over 25 years, a major concern in the study of nidation. It has been the challenge of trying to explain the basis of receptivity and its transience that has provoked many, if not all, of the studies embodied in this symposium. More recently, as Dr. Psychoyos related, the knowledge of the endocrine basis of receptivity has allowed development of a promising agent, the antiprogestogen RU 486, which may be used to manipulate the endocrine balance in order to prevent implantation or, conceivably (pun intentional), to allow implantation after, for example, asynchronous embryo transfer.

Dr. Mead's study of the endocrine climate necessary to support implantation in mustelids has indicated that even at the endocrine level our knowledge is still incomplete. It appears that a requirement for progesterone in the establishment of receptivity is common to all placental mammals, but Dr. Mead had shown clearly that some animals require at least one other ovarian factor to induce implantation. It has been argued persuasively, in a recent review,[2] that estradiol, whatever the source, ovarian or embryonic, is required in all species. Dr. Mead's findings indicate, however, that neither estradiol nor androstenedione suffice, and some other luteal factor is essential in addition to progesterone. One may speculate that the unknown factor is nevertheless a steroid, perhaps of an unfamiliar sort. Certainly unusual steroids are produced by some species. Aside from the already familiar equine estrogens, there is the unusual 19-norandostenedione, which has recently been identified as a major constituent of porcine follicular fluid.[3]

The idea that hitherto unfamiliar steroids may be involved in nidation is implicit in the work of Dr. Dey, whose thesis is that conversion of estradiol to a catechol estrogen is critical for implantation induction. The reported effects of catechol estrogens on prostaglandin formation[4] and the synergism with histamine in nidation are exciting and welcome to an associate of Shelesnyak who has been involved with the histamine theory of decidual induction. It is therefore also noteworthy that the mouse blastocyst has been shown to be capable of producing both the histamine[5] and the catechol estrogens[6] that qualify these substances as the putative embryonic signals initiating nidation, at least until more conclusive information is obtained. The histamine involved in nidation thus would not come from mast cells, as we noted some years ago[7] and that was pointed out again more recently with the finding that decidualization occurs normally in the uteri of genetically mast cell-deficient mice.[8]

Implicit in the demonstration that an estrogen, having high uterotrophic activity but impaired convertibility to catechols, does not induce implantation in ovariectomized rats is the concept of an extragenomic mode of estrogen action. This is not a new alternative to the generally accepted mechanism involving interaction at the transcriptional level. Clara Szego attacked the idea that the primary locus of estradiol action is at the level of the genome some 20 years ago,[9] just at the time that transcription and translational responses were the latest topics of study. More recently, extragenomic actions gained more importance when it was found that actinomycin D and cycloheximide, drugs that inhibit, respectively, transcription and translation, only partially prevent some of the uterine responses to estradiol.[10,11] Similarly, estradiol-induced activation of the blastocyst is not prevented by actinomycin D,[12] although later processes that involve RNA and DNA synthesis are inhibited.[13]

Dr. Yochim's work also implicates an extragenomic path in estrogen action, in the shifting of endometrial metabolism towards preparation for cell division. We were reminded that in the rat, as in the mouse, a wave of stromal proliferation not only precedes uterine receptivity but is essential to its establishment. If this proliferation is prevented by agents that, although not inhibitors of DNA synthesis, shift the equilibrium of the NAD kinase—glycohydrolase system away from the salvage pathway—then decidualization is impaired.

Now, the point of my dwelling on extragenomic pathways and stromal proliferation is that the proliferation can be induced without estrogen. In species such as the guinea pig and rabbit, there is no appreciable estrogen present during progestation when stromal proliferation occurs, although uterine edema that is presumably a response to earlier, estrous estrogen is present.

The presence of edema as a prelude to stromal proliferation seems to be a common feature suggesting that the two phenomena are related, perhaps due to the pressure generated by the edema. An indication that this is indeed the case is that distension of the uterus by intraluminal injection of oil or saline, causing a pressure analogous to that produced by edema, in ovariectomized mice primed with estrogen and then treated with progesterone, elicits intense mitotic activity in the stroma.[14] In the nonprogestational uterus, distension causes only epithelial proliferation.[15] Thus it appears that in the case of estrogen action on the uterus, proliferative responses are the result of the edema rather than nuclear interactions with the steroid, and progesterone shifts the reaction to the mechanical stimulus from the epithelium to the stroma. Dr. Yochim's elucidation and exposition of the β-nicotinamide adenine dinucleotide (NAD) system's responses to various stimuli provide an elegant explanation of how mechanical stimuli may suppress NAD phosphate (NADP) formation and favor the salvage pathway leading to DNA synthesis and mitosis.

Although it remains to be determined whether mechanically induced stromal proliferation confers receptivity on the uterus, one may hypothesize that the ability of traumatic stimuli to induce decidualization in the absence of estrogenic stimulation is the consequence of the ability of trauma to first induce a proliferative response, and by virtue of lingering stimulation due to the trauma, also provide the decidual induction stimulus to a now sensitized uterus. Trauma would thus have two distinct actions: sensitization and induction.

Because this hypothesis presumes persistence of the stimulus to be necessary, it was with particular interest that I listened to Dr. Kennedy's account of the requirement for an extended infusion or prolonged action of prostaglandin (PG) in the induction of decidualization. An additional reason for the interest, particularly for those of us who have been supporters of the histamine theory of decidual induction, is the association of PGs with histamine in many systems. In fact, new vigor for the histamine theory, in addition to that supplied by Dr. Dey, is provided by the extent to which histamine and, particularly, PGE$_2$ are agonists of each other. It has been shown that prostaglandins have little intrinsic ability to induce edema, but rather, synergize with other substances such as histamine or bradykinine.[16] Also, PGs appear to be involved in the release of histamine and may be released with it.[17] Another possibility that Dr. Kennedy's work suggests is that prolonged infusion of PG, perhaps in combination with histamine, will overcome the perplexing refractoriness of the deepitheliated uterus to decidual induction.[18]

Turning our attention to the epithelium, we have some very topical presentations (again, pun intentional). The surface epithelium of the uterus is still very much an enigma. We know a great deal about it without having any understanding of how it performs its function as a signal transmitter or transducer. A recent relevant finding indicates that epithelial responses to estrogen are dependent on direct contact with the stroma, the latter somehow conditioning or instructing the epithelium to respond characteristically.[19] It would be reasonable that the reverse relation also holds, that is, that characteristic differentiation of the stroma in response to exogenous stimuli is dependent on some influence of the epithelium, as suggested above[18] and also by the *in vitro* model Dr. Weitlauf described to us. We may look to such *in vitro* studies to unravel the nature of the influences of each tissue on the other. Nevertheless, we certainly need more information of the epithelium's internal functions, that is, functions occurring independently of the stroma. The papers by Dr. Moulton and Dr. Parr represent the vanguard of the attack on the knotty problem of just what it is that the epithelium does for the endometrium in preparation for nidation (despite the fact that the uterus, after getting what it needs from epithelium, then ungratefully discards it!).

Dr. Moulton's work is a major step towards an understanding of at least some of the ways in which the transmitter/transducer functions are performed, providing the first biochemical rationale for such function in uterine receptivity. If the limited ability of the methylation inhibitor, 3-deazaadenosine (3-DZA), to inhibit decidual induction is due to its short half-life and brief action, then we have here another demonstration of the essential persistence of the induction message. It should be noted that a likely relevant action of 3-DZA, in addition to inhibition of methyl transferase, is the inhibition of the release of PGs and histamine associated with phospholipid methylation.[20]

The work of the Parrs has shown us that traffic across the epithelium is bidirectional, and there is selective transport of macromolecules into the uterine lumen. The finding that such movement is augmented by hormonal preparation of the uterus for nidation suggests a functional relation, but other than influencing the blastocyst, the role of this transport of materials is obscure.

Now we come to the result of all the efforts of the uterus (and of the investigators): the decidua itself. Two of today's presentations focused on cellular aspects of immunity involving the decidua. Previously, the role of decidualization as an immunological barrier, sequestering the implanting embryo from being fingered and protecting it from cruising hit-men (to stretch a metaphor) has been considered mainly from a phenomenological basis rather than, as in this symposium, on a cytological basis. Dr. Tachi's studies on uterine macrophages assign to the decidua the role of blocking access to the embryonic allograft of besieging macrophages and immune effector cells, thereby preventing both recognition and attack.

Dr. Lala's presentation complemented that of Dr. Tachi, exploring the nature of the cells constituting the decidua and which contribute to its immunoprotective function at later stages of gestation. A major feature of this work is the indication that a subset of lymphoid decidual cells exerts a protective action by releasing PGE_2, which in turn suppresses activation and proliferation of killer cells. Dr. Lala's identification of the lymphoid cells as derived from bone marrow, however, is somewhat controversial, at least with regard to quantitative contribution to the decidual cell population and has been challenged by investigators who claim that bone marrow-derived cells constitute, at most, a very small proportion of decidual cells.[21,22] Nevertheless, the residence of even small numbers of immunocompetent cells in the uterine stroma indicates that an immunological reaction as the initial recognition of the presence of the embryo, which we proposed some years ago,[1] is not a very far-fetched idea. Another recent finding suggestive of such a reaction is the readier implantation of blastocysts transferred into pseudopregnant rats when the recipients are stimulated by intravaginal insemination on the day before the transfer,[23] the stimulus presumably attracting infiltration of the uterus by lymphocytes.

In discussing the work presented today, I have asked some questions without expecting immediate answers. Some of the answers would depend on a means of observing the course of decidualization in the absence of distracting, but essential, influences of the supporting tissues. In the past, we thought that the pseudopregnant animal provided an admirable model, free of the complications of embryonic participation in decidualization. In some respects now, all of the animal except for the stroma may be considered extraneous with respect to poststimulation changes. Dr. Leavitt appears to be a convert to that view, offering us a means of eliminating all but the irreducible decidual cell itself, in culture. Not only has he shown us the means of growing the differentiated cell in culture, but he has also identified for us the cell-specific markers that are indispensable in recognizing the decidual cell in culture. The culture system and the marker proteins will be of inestimable value in helping to unravel the sequence of changes in decidual differentiation at the molecular level and enable recognition of decidual induction *in vitro*, when that breakthrough is achieved.

The remaining paper, presented by Dr. Lejeune, though not last in order of delivery, caps the other papers, after a fashion, by dealing with what may be the principal, if not sole, justification for our efforts, applicability to humans. It was gratifying, therefore, to learn that clinical experience shows uterine receptivity in the human to parallel that in our favorite subjects, the rat and mouse, exhibiting the same hormonal dependency and similarly narrow window for embryo transplantation.

Having commented, however briefly, on the papers presented (being limited both by time and my facility with the particular focus of the respective papers) I should remind you of my intention, at Dr. Shelesnyak's invitation, to update the 1970 model of theoretical bases for uterine sensitization and decidualization. In order to justify the model's premises, it is necessary to review the principal evidence, beginning with work from Shelesnyak's own laboratory and summarized in FIGURE 1.

First and most intriguing was the demonstration of the restricted period of uterine responsiveness to decidual induction found using intraperitoneally administered pyrathiazine.[24] This now-familiar window is only 12–14 hours wide at half-maximal response (curve R, shaded). The search for correlates of this short-lived sensitivity led to the finding that total uterine DNA also increased temporarily[25] (curve A) and that both the sensitivity and increase in DNA are dependent on prior estrogen action.[25,26] These findings placed on a firm footing the concept of the "estrogen surge",[27,28] vindicated since then by direct measurement of serum estradiol levels.[29]

Investigation of cell dynamics thought to underlie the association between increased DNA levels and receptivity revealed that a period of intense stromal mitotic activity followed "surge" estrogen action and both preceded and produced the state of receptivity (curve B).[1,30,31] Other studies revealed that the proliferative pool can be depleted, resulting in impaired receptivity in the subsequent progestation.[1,32] Reestablishment of the pool occurs as the result of several cycles of proliferation occurring at successive estruses (shown in the model of FIGURE 2 in the vertical sequence at the left). Interference with

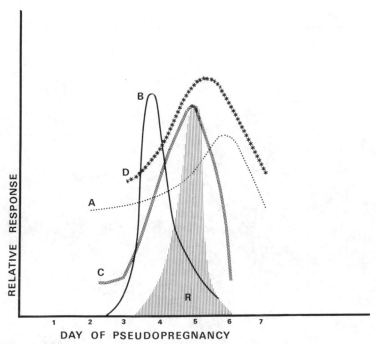

FIGURE 1. Summary of evidence on which the model is based. Shaded curve, R: decidual response to stimulation at different times;[24] curve A: total uterine DNA;[25] curve B: stromal mitotic activity;[31] curve C: rate of DNA synthesis ([3H]thymidine incorporation per horn);[30] curve D: mean Feulgen DNA per stromal cell nucleus.[37]

the wave of proliferation by other means, as described by Dr. Yochim,[33] likewise impairs the decidual response. These observations suggest that the degree of uterine sensitivity is related to the number of stromal cells dividing during progestation.

Consideration of the temporal relation between DNA levels and mitotic activity indicated, however, that the DNA level continued to rise after the cessation of mitosis, until receptivity peaked, and declined only thereafter. These and other findings were integrated in the 1970 model and led to the postulate that receptivity was established by the formation of a metastable subpopulation of stromal cells committed to differentiation directly into decidual cells if stimulated, or to degenerate and die if not. The loss of these predecidual cells would thus account for the loss of sensitivity and for the decline in DNA levels.

This postulate remains a central feature of the current model (FIG. 2) and has been strengthened by more recent studies. Several workers have shown that peak DNA synthesis in the pseudopregnant rat uterus occurs after the mitotic peak is passed and coincides with maximal uterine sensitivity

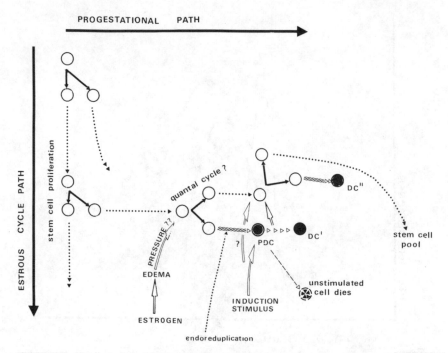

FIGURE 2. Theoretical model of mechanisms in establishment of uterine receptivity and decidualization. PDC: predecidual cell, formed from quantal mitosis of stromal cell; DC': primary decidual cell, formed directly from stimulated PDC; DC": secondary decidual cell, formed by transformation of product of quantal mitosis induced in stromal cell secondarily to decidual induction stimulation.

(FIG. 1, curve C),[30,34] most of the label being found in the subepithelial stroma, from which the primary decidual cells arise. The postmitotic DNA synthesis is not always noted if incorporation is calculated on the basis of changes in specific activity of uterine DNA rather than as total incorporation, and therefore the peak may not be found at the time of maximal sensitivity.[35,36] Leroy and Galand[37] found, however, that the mean nuclear content of DNA in stromal cells reached a maximum after the stromal mitotic index declined but at the time of peak uterine receptivity (FIG. 1, curve D).

More recent studies, in the mouse[38] and in the rat,[39] have confirmed the postulated existence of two populations of stromal cells. One, a small population, located subepithelially and mesometrially, undergoes hormone-induced mitosis on day 3 of progestation (open circles in the horizontal sequence, the progestational path in the model) and continues to synthesize DNA (twined line leading to cell-labeled PDC in model) and, in response to induction, transforms without division into decidual cells (solid circle labeled DC') forming the periluminal, primary decidual zone. The second, a major stromal population, located to the periphery of the subepithelial population and extending to the myometrial border, undergoes little proliferation in response to the strogen surge, but proliferates during decidualization after the primary decidual zone differentiates. The proliferative response of this major stromal population spreads radially and is followed by differentiation into decidual cells, except for the most basally located cells, which remain untransformed and are the source for repopulation of the stroma in the recovery of the uterus after gestation or experimental decidualization. This is indicated in the model at the upper right by the arrows connecting open circles and leading to the circle (cell) marked DC" and by the dotted line leading down to the right.

In summary, the model embodies the postulates that during successive estrous cycles, some stromal cells proliferate, building up a pool that during progestation responds to estrogen stimulation (by way of a pressure stimulus) with asymmetric mitosis (a quantal division,[40] proposed in the model of O'Grady and Bell[36]). Endoreduplication then occurs in some of the daughter cells in the subepithelial, antimesometrial region, forming predecidual cells (PDC in the model) that confer receptivity on the uterus and respond to stimulation by immediate differentiation into the primary decidual cells. This rapidity of response without an intervening mitosis would be due to the condition of endopolyploidy, which allows the increased RNA synthesis necessary for differentiation but is suppressed during mitosis (see Nagl[41] for a discussion of the significance of endoreduplication in differentiation). If unstimulated, the PDC degenerate, and the ability of the uterus to respond to induction stimulation is lost. Deciduogenic stimuli, while inducing transformation of the PDC, also initiate quantal mitosis in the stroma adjacent to the PDC, the response spreading radially, perhaps propagated by the edema, which is also an early response to decidual induction. It appears that the ability of cells to differentiate into decidual cells is dependent on prior quantal mitosis, one daughter cell then reinitiating DNA synthesis as a prelude to differentiation.

This model offers an explanation of the effectiveness of traumatic stimuli in inducing decidualization outside the period of receptivity by way of induction of quantal mitosis that then provides the requisite sensitivity.

I hope this model raises new questions as well as offers postulates that are amenable to testing. The nature of the interactions between the stroma and epithelium, the molecular basis of decidual induction, and the identity of the signals and intermediating messengers all remain challenges. The research presented today shows that we are well on the way to meeting them.

Let us hope that these will no longer be challenges at the next symposium on nidation. I look forward to the new challenges that will then be offered to us.

REFERENCES

1. SHELESNYAK, M. C. & G. J. MARCUS. 1970. Steroidal conditioning of the endometrium for nidation. Adv. Bioscience 6: 303-313.
2. LEVASSEUR, M.-C. 1984. The involvement of estradiol at the time of implantation in placental mammals. Anim. Reprod. Sci. 7: 467-488.
3. KHALIL, M. W. 1984. Identification of 19-nor-4-androstene-3,17-dione (19-norandrostenedione) as a major steroid in porcine follicular fluid. Proc. 7th Int. Congr. Endocrinol. Excerpta Medica Int. Congr. Ser. 652: Abstr. 1011.
4. KELLY, R. W. & M. H. ABEL. 1980. In Advances in Prostaglandin and Thromboxane Research. B. Samuelsson, P. W. Ramwell & R. Paoletti, Eds. Vol. 8: 1369-1370. Raven Press. New York.
5. DEY, S. K. & D. C. JOHNSON. 1980. Histamine formation by mouse preimplantation embryos. J. Reprod. Fertil. 60: 457-460.
6. HOVERSLAND, R. C. 1985. Presence of 2-/4-estradiol hydrolase in mouse embryos collected on day 5 of pregnancy. Biol. Reprod. 32 (Suppl. 1) Abstr. 205.
7. MARCUS, G. J. 1969. In Ovum Implantation. M. C. Shelesnyak & G. J. Marcus, Eds.: 80. Gordon & Breach. New York.
8. HATANAKA, K., Y. KITAMURA, K. MAEYAMA, T. WATANABE & K. MATSUMOTO. 1983. Deciduoma formation in uterus of genetically mast cell-deficient W/Wᵛ mice. Biol. Reprod. 27: 25-28.
9. SZEGO, C. M. & B. LIPPE. 1965. Mediation by adrenocortical hypersecretion of the suppressive influence of actinomycin D on (rat) uterine estrogen sensitivity. Steroids (Suppl. II) 235-247.
10. LEROY, F., C. BOGAERT & J. VAN HOECK. 1975. Inactivité de la cycloheximide sur certains effets des stéroides ovariens responsables du conditionnement de l'utérus à la nidation. C.R. Acad. Sci. 281: 2005-2007.
11. LEROY, F., J. VAN HOECK & C. BOGAERT. 1976. Inability of actinomycin D to act upon the uterine refractory state resulting from nidatory oestrogen action in rats. J. Endocrinol. 68: 137-140.
12. FINN, C. A. 1974. The induction of implantation in mice by actinomycin D. J. Endocrinol. 60: 199-200.
13. BURIN, P. & P. SARTOR. 1965. Inhibition de la réaction déciduale par l'actinomycin D. C. R. Soc. Biol. (Paris) 159: 141-144.
14. MARCUS, G. J. Unpublished work.
15. BIGSBY, R. M. & G. R. CUNHA. 1985. Progesterone inhibition of uterine epithelial cell proliferation does not involve estrogen receptor mechanism. Proc. 67th Meeting Endocr. Soc. Abstr. 204.
16. WILLIAMS, T. J. & M. J. PECK. 1977. Role of prostaglandin-mediated vasodilatation in inflammation. Nature (London) 270: 530-532.
17. MAGRO, A. M. 1982. Effects of inhibitors of arachidonic acid metabolism upon IgE and non-IgE-mediated histamine release. Int. J. Immunopharmacol. 4: 15-20.
18. LEJEUNE, B., J. VAN HOECK & F. LEROY. 1981. Transmitter role of the luminal uterine epithelium in the induction of decidualization in rats. J. Reprod. Fertil. 61: 235-240.
19. COOKE, P. S., D. K. FUJII, F.-D. A. UCHIMA, L. I. SEWELL, H. A. BERN & G. R. CUNHA. 1985. Restoration of normal morphology and function in cultured vaginal and uterine epithelium transplanted with stroma in vivo. Proc. 67th Meeting Endocr. Soc. Abstr. 260.
20. HIRATA, F. & J. AXELROD. 1980. Phospholipid methylation and biological signal transmission. Science 209: 1082-1090.

21. GAMBEL, P., J. ROSSANT, R. D. HUNZIKER & T. G. WEGMANN. 1985. Origin of decidual
     cells in murine pregnancy and pseudopregnancy. Transplantation **39:** 443-445.
22. FOWLIS, D. J. & J. D. ANSELL. 1985. Evidence that decidual cells are not derived from
     bone marrow. Transplantation **39:** 445-446.
23. CARP, H., H. ORNSTEIN, S. MASHIACH & L. NEBEL. 1984. Implantation of transferred
     blastocysts: influence of insemination in rats. Isr. J. Med. Sci. **20:** 6545 (Abstr.).
24. SHELESNYAK, M. C. & P. F. KRAICER. 1961. A physiological method for inducing
     decidualization of the rat uterus: standardization and evaluation. J. Reprod. Fertil. **2:**
     438-446.
25. SHELESNYAK, M. C. & L. TIC. 1963. Studies on the mechanism of nidation. IV. Synthetic
     processes in the decidualizing uterus. Acta Endocrinol. **42:** 465-472.
26. SHELESNYAK, M. C. & L. TIC. 1963. Studies on the mechanism of nidation. V. Suppression
     of synthetic processes of the uterus (DNA, RNA and protein) following inhibition of
     decidualization by an anti-oestrogen, ethanoxytriphetol (MER-25). Acta Endocrinol. **43:**
     462-468.
27. SHELESNYAK, M. C., P. F. KRAICER & G. H. ZEILMAKER. 1963. Studies on the mechanism
     of nidation. I. The oestrogen surge of pseudopregnancy and prográvidity and its role in
     the process of decidualization. Acta Endocrinol. **42:** 225-232.
28. SHELESNYAK, M. C. & P. F. KRAICER. 1960. Décidualisation: une étude expérimentale.
     Extrait du colloque: Les fonctions de nidation utérine et leur troubles. 87-101. Masson
     et Cie. Paris.
29. WATSON, J., F. B. ANDERSON, M. ALAM, J. E. O'GRADY & P. J. HEALD. 1975. Plasma
     hormones and pituitary luteinising hormone in the rat during the early states of pregnancy
     and following post coital treatment with tamoxifen ICI 46,474. J. Endocrinol. **65:** 7-17.
30. TACHI, C., S. TACHI & H. R. LINDNER. 1972. Modification by progesterone of oestradiol-
     induced cell proliferation, RNA synthesis and oestradiol distribution in the rat uterus.
     J. Reprod. Fertil. **31:** 59-76.
31. MARCUS, G. J. 1974. Mitosis in the rat uterus during the estrous cycle, early pregnancy
     and early pseudopregnancy. Biol. Reprod. **10:** 447-452.
32. MARCUS, G. J. 1970. A cellular basis for implantation failure due to massive decidualization
     in the rat. Proc. 3rd Meeting Soc. Stud. Reprod. Abstr. 46.
33. YOCHIM, J. M. 1984. Modulation of uterine sensitivity to decidual induction in the rat by
     nicotinamide: challenge and extension of a model of progestational differentiation. Biol.
     Reprod. **30:** 637-645.
34. HEALD, P. J., J. E. O'GRADY, A. O'HARE & M. VASS. 1975. Nucleic acid metabolism of
     cells of the luminal epithelium and stroma of the rat uterus during early pregnancy. J.
     Reprod. Fertil. **45:** 129-138.
35. O'GRADY, J. E. & P. J. HEALD. 1976. Uterine nucleic acid and phospholipid metabolism
     in the early stages of pregnancy. J. Endocrinol. **68:** 33 p.
36. O'GRADY, J. E. & S. C. BELL. 1977. The role of the endometrium in blastocyst implantation.
     In Development in Mammals. M. H. Johnson, Ed. Vol. **1:** 165-243. Elsevier/North
     Holland. Amsterdam.
37. LEROY, F. & P. GALAND. 1970. Activité du DNA dans l'endomètre de la rate pseudo-
     gestante pendant la phase de réceptivité. *In* Ovo-Implantation Human Gonadotropins
     and Prolactin. P. O. Hubinont, F. Leroy, C. Roybn & P. Leleux, Eds.: 130-138. Karger.
     Basel.
38. DAS, R. M. & L. MARTIN. 1978. Uterine DNA synthesis and cell proliferation during
     early decidualization induced by oil in mice. J. Reprod. Fertil. **53:** 125-128.
39. KLEINFELD, R. G. & J. D. O'SHEA. 1983. Spatial and temporal patterns of deoxyribonucleic
     acid synthesis and mitosis in the endometrial stroma during decidualization in the pseu-
     dopregnant rat. Biol. Reprod. **28:** 691-702.
40. HOLTZER, H. & N. RUBINSTEIN. 1977. Binary decisions, quantal cells cycles and cell
     diversification. *In* Cell Differentiation in Microorganizma, Plants and Animals. L. Nover
     & K. Mothes, Eds.: 512. Elsevier/North Holland. Amsterdam.
41. NAGL, W. 1978. Endopolyploidy and Polyteny in Differentiation and Evolution. Elsevier/
     North Holland. Amsterdam.

Index of Contributors